Beyond the Blindness

Beyond the Blindness

My Story of Losing Sight and Living Life

Ted Hinson

ISBN-13: 9781548252052
ISBN-10: 1548252050
Library of Congress Control Number: 2017909843
CreateSpace Independent Publishing Platform
North Charleston, South Carolina

Acknowledgments

I would like to thank my good friends Jim Langdon, Matt O'Meilia and Laurie Tilley for not only offering their professional expertise—as a publisher, copywriter and marketing executive, respectively—but also for providing valuable opinions, ideas and overall support. Their efforts made this book better.

And, thank you to Langdon Publishing graphic designer Georgia Brooks for creating the book's cover, and editor Judy Langdon for proofreading the manuscript.

Table of contents

Acknowledgments··v
Foreword ···ix
Prologue ···xi

1   A "Permanent" Diagnosis ··························· 1
2   Beginnings ····································· 6
3   Acceptance ···································· 9
4   The Rookie································14
5   Rehab Me ······································ 22
6   Game Changer ······························29
7   More Than Man's Best Friend ··················33
8   Getting Traction································ 44
9   A Bite Out of Life·····························52
10 My Normal·································· 66
11 A Bigger Loss ·······························75
12 The Family Way ····························· 84
13 Not The Final Chapter·······················87

About the Author ····························95

Foreword

By Jim Stovall

Thirty years ago, I received what I thought at the time was the worst news possible. I was diagnosed with a condition that would result in my blindness. Since that time, I have learned that there are a myriad of things much worse than being blind, but it takes a bit of experience and some good examples to grasp that.

I have long believed that we should never take advice from anyone who doesn't have what we want, nor should we take directions from anyone who hasn't been where we want to go.

Ted Hinson lost his sight about the time I did. Although he didn't know it at the time, in many ways he became my guide, mentor, and an example of what I could be. I followed a path that led me to be an author, speaker, executive, movie producer, and the owner of a television network. This was a long road, and for many years, I had little or nothing to show for my efforts.

Ted took a more conventional path and began climbing the corporate ladder and succeeding in the business world. As a blind person, he launched into the very competitive energy industry where he became known for being reliable and dependable. As I was struggling to find my way, many people told me they had run into this blind guy named Ted Hinson and his guide dog in the downtown business district of the city where we live. Since I didn't seem to be going anywhere, people used Ted's example as a way to both challenge and encourage me.

Decades later, I finally achieved some success of my own, and I have people around the world who read my books and contact me. Many of these people are blind or know someone who is blind, and they are looking for advice and direction. Often, they can't relate to me as an author, speaker, and businessperson, so I tell them about my friend Ted Hinson who, under difficult circumstances, built a successful career and became a great husband to his wife and father to his children.

I am in the message business, and I try to share hope, encouragement, and possibilities with those who hear me speak, read my books, or watch my movies. I tell stories about success, but Ted Hinson, in many ways, is the embodiment of my message. In spite of circumstances that would derail or destroy most people, Ted has created a life, a family, and a career that anyone would aspire to.

Within these pages, you are going to meet a man who has no sight but can share vision and perspective with you. I hope you will do what I did and simply follow the leader to your own destiny.

Prologue

On a cloud-swept winter afternoon in 1987, the Cadillac weaved in spasmodic, crab-like movements down a lonely country road that sliced straight through seemingly endless wheat fields of russet stubble. The car, perhaps fortunately, had no one to marvel at its strange behavior that frigid day.

Earlier that morning, the Hinson family, including Aquina and Grant Buehrig, Ted's sister and brother-in-law, had gathered in romantic-sounding but visually isolated Roseland, a pin point of houses in a distant corner of Kansas. To underscore the hamlet's remoteness, the arrival of the Hinson clan for the traditional Christmas holiday with Ted's and Aquina's maternal grandmother, Minnie Aquino, arguably doubled the population of this tiny community of mostly Italian immigrants and their relatives.

After a dinner that always included as much spaghetti as turkey, Ted and Grant talked about Ted's new life and what he missed most since his sudden loss of sight the prior year. Ted looked at Grant and decided it was getting behind the wheel again.

And I decided why not? I drove the two of us to a spot on what looked like a nearly forgotten strip of macadam about a half mile away. There, Ted settled into the driver's seat. We launched down the road, Ted steering confidently with his eyes looking ahead, and I, shouting apprehensively with my heart in my mouth, "Left, left, right, right!"

This simple journey exemplified Ted's inner strength and courage that would carry him down the more tortuous path life had laid before him. In the

30 or so years since then, Aquina and I not once have heard Ted utter a single word of complaint or remorse. Ted not only accepted his new challenge, but took it on with wholehearted resolve. Buoyed by the conviction of his faith, Ted's attitude has always been to persevere and to make the most of what life offers for himself and his family.

Let's face it—I think we all wonder how we would cope. This uncertainty in ourselves is in part what ironically makes Ted so extraordinary. Ted's overarching optimism, his strength of character, and his insights into what matters most are distinguishing attributes that I know we all acknowledge and admire.

I believe good comes to all of us who know Ted and learn from his positive example. Aquina and I will always be grateful to Ted for what he has taught us about life's priorities. Ted has shown us how to put setbacks into perspective and to realize that happiness, and not perfection, is perhaps one of life's most important goals.

Grant Buehrig
Reston, Virginia

1

A "Permanent" Diagnosis

Dr. Brad Farris is a good man—caring, thoughtful, knowledgeable and possessing a good bedside manner.

"I'm sorry, Ted, but your blindness is permanent," said Dr. Farris.

"Permanent?" I responded.

"Yes. Now that the inflammation has gone down, we can see . . . it's apparent that the optic nerves are damaged. The tissue should be a pink and healthy color, but yours is a light, grayish color, meaning that it's dead."

"What can we do now?" I asked. "What's the remedy? A nerve transplant or some sort of rejuvenation—something like that?"

"No, you can't transplant this type of nerve tissue," he explained. "It would be like reconnecting all the thousands of fiber endings of a rope that's been cut—just not possible. Science has not had any luck with transplanting or rejuvenating dead nerve tissue yet, at least not this type of tissue. The optic nerve tissue is very similar to the spinal cord tissue. When they start having success with transplanting, reattaching or rejuvenating spinal cord tissue, I think we might have some luck with doing the same with optic nerve tissue."

The above conversation took place in July 1986. Six months earlier, I was a petroleum landman working for a large and successful oil and gas company in Oklahoma City. A landman is the person who goes to the county courthouse and reviews title documents to identify the owner of a particular tract of land where geologists have located underlying minerals (oil, gas, etc.). After identifying the title ownership, the landman contacts these mineral owners to negotiate an oil and gas lease. Once the company has secured the lease, the company has the rights to drill on this land.

In January 1986, I was 27 years old and business was getting tough. The price of oil was dropping fast, and when the price of your product no longer economically justifies your company's cost of producing it—drilling oil and gas wells, in our case—then production halts. The land work necessary to drill wells also stops, which means there's little need for a landman.

So, that month, our company had a round of layoffs. Everyone was called into the office in downtown Oklahoma City. Being relatively young, professionally immature and naive, I had no idea of the purpose of this all-inclusive meeting. I doubt I even knew what the price of oil was at that time.

In the meeting, my name was not called, which meant my job was safe. This was my first experience with the dreaded phenomenon of corporate downsizing. My second came two months later, in March, and this time I was not so lucky. Like many others, I got the axe, a casualty of $9-a-barrel oil.

I had worked at this company for three years and thoroughly enjoyed it. I met many good hardworking, fun guys with much in common—all starting families, playing company softball, having had similar college experiences. I felt this was the place for me, and was confident a good, promising future was ahead of me, my wife and young son. But at 27, I was too naïve to think about things beyond my control, like the fluctuating price of oil and natural gas, that can throw life a huge curveball.

My wife, Pat, a schoolteacher, was not making enough to support us long-term, but with my severance package and frugal spending, we felt we'd be okay until I found a new position, however and wherever I could.

Over the next two or three weeks, I got on the job hunt. I knew a guy who knew a guy in Tulsa who called me for an interview. It wasn't for an oil and gas land position, but a job similar enough to qualify me for a face-to-face meeting. During my drive to Tulsa from Oklahoma City for this interview, I noticed some of the street signs seemed a little blurry. I figured I needed to clean my contact lenses when I got back that night. Maybe it was time for an eye test and new correction on the lenses. No big deal.

The next day, things were a little more blurry. So, the following day I went to the optometrist for an eye check. During the exam, the doctor said something looked odd and suggested I go to an ophthalmologist for a more thorough exam.

The next day seemed a little worse.

I got into the ophthalmologist and went through several tests, checking for brightness and darkness, peripheral vision, tunnel vision and about any type of eyeball test imaginable. At this point, I could tell by the doctor's expression and voice he was perplexed and concerned. "Do you have someone to drive you home?" he asked. I told him I could drive myself. He looked at me and said, "I don't think that's a very good idea."

Well, I did drive myself home, and as I did I recall thinking, "This is not a very good idea."

The next day was worse.

Oklahoma City's Dean McGee Eye Institute is a nationally renowned facility specializing in every type of eye problem. I was fortunate to get an appointment there the week after my visit with the ophthalmologist. By then, however, my sight was gone. My wife and I had no idea what was going on and what the cause could be.

Dr. Farris, a neuro-ophthalmologist, recently had been recruited to Dean McGee. I was one of his first patients in his new position at the Institute. He seemed on top of all things related to vision problems, so I felt I was in the right place. He immediately scheduled every type of diagnostic test imaginable: X-rays, blood work, an MRI, spinal tap, EEG—you name it. These tests were conducted over the next couple of weeks. Until all tests were completed and the final results were provided to Dr. Farris, we would not know the cause or, more important, the prognosis. So, we waited.

Finally, all test results came in and were reviewed by Dr. Farris and the staff at Dean McGee. Pat and I were called in for a consultation. This was late May 1986, about a month after our initial visit.

"Ted, all tests came back normal," said Dr. Farris. "Nothing seems out of the ordinary and I don't know what additional tests we could do to look for anything else. I think your loss of sight is temporary, probably caused from the stress of losing your job."

"But I don't remember feeling all stressed out over losing my job," I said.

"You can't tell me you didn't feel stress over losing your job. You have a wife, a baby, a mortgage. This is a stressful situation; we've seen this kind of thing before, usually related to a military situation in the battlefield. The body can do some weird things when it experiences stress and shock."

"So, just temporary?" I asked, feeling somewhat relieved.

"Yes, so just go home and relax," Dr. Farris said.

"Go home and relax?"

"Ok, I know it sounds easy enough, but go home and try to relax and we'll get you back in here every couple of weeks for checkups."

We did go in every two weeks, but there were no changes. My sight had dimmed to only a little light perception, so I could faintly tell light from dark—nothing useable, but better than total black, I thought.

About two months later, Dr. Farris noticed the tissue damage mentioned earlier. He diagnosed it as optic neuritis. I understood it as most likely being some sort of virus that had settled in the optic nerves—very rare, especially because it affected both optic nerves. He explained that the eyeballs act as cameras, transmitting images through the optic nerves to the back of the brain, which identifies the picture. The dead optic nerve tissue created a block that prohibited transmission from the eyes to the brain.

Dr. Farris asked if I remember possibly being in contact with some harsh chemicals, such as fertilizer. He said this could affect some types of nerve tissue. I couldn't think of any such contact.

So, there we were. He'd done all he could do. I told Dr. Farris that I felt I owed it to myself to get a second opinion—nothing personal. He understood. I realized the damaged tissue was probably irreversible, but I needed to have someone else take a look, review the medical records and tests just to be certain nothing else could be done. I had a sister in the Washington, D.C., area, so it seemed the Johns Hopkins Hospital in Baltimore was a good option for this second opinion.

A month later I was at Johns Hopkins. Same results, same diagnosis, and confirmation that Dr. Farris and Dean McGee had done all things possible, diagnosed the optic neuritis properly and nothing else could have been done.

"A rare, rare case," concluded the physicians at Johns Hopkins.

"Not quite rare enough," I thought to myself as we left to return to Tulsa. Now what?

2

Beginnings

I grew up in Tulsa, Oklahoma, the youngest of three kids and the only boy. I'd say we were smack in the middle of middle class. My parents both worked, we lived in a nice, easy neighborhood, in a clean, simple house, and had everything we needed.

Neither of my parents, Ted and Jody Hinson, went to college, so sending their kids to college was very important to them. I graduated from Edison High School in 1977, in a good class with many friends. I played basketball all through school. Edison had a tradition of successful basketball teams and many talented players. I was what a coach would label "a good practice player," meaning I was tall enough and athletic enough to make the team, but I shouldn't expect much game time.

Our basketball team was much like a club: you had to work hard to get in, work hard to be accepted and learn to take the good with the bad. Like any club, we built strong bonds and developed lifelong friendships. During my junior and senior seasons, we advanced through the state Class 4A playoffs and made it to the championship game. We lost in the finals both years, but the success we achieved and the resulting war stories are still lied about today.

I went on to the University of Oklahoma, the only college I ever wanted to attend. I was an average high school student and attending college was something I always wanted to do—not so much for the purpose of increasing my intellect as it was for the friends I expected to gain and fun I expected to have. I assumed that by simply being in an academic environment, the education part would magically take care of itself. Not the focus a guy needs when beginning college, I know, but at least I was smart enough to understand that a college degree would come in handy someday.

I joined the Alpha Tau Omega (ATO) fraternity. It was a good frat (does anybody ever say they were in a bad fraternity?), a strong house that had several campus leaders and lots of pre-law and pre-med brothers. But primarily it was lots of stupid fun and many good, solid guys who became lifelong friends. If you can't survive a little stupidity, you never learn exactly how lucky you are, and exactly what not to do again. That's all I really need to say on that subject.

During my sophomore year I began dating Pat Berry, who was also a sophomore. She was from Henryetta, a small Oklahoma town about an hour south of Tulsa. As a big city boy from Tulsa, I knew I could teach her a thing or two—not exactly. Pat was much more focused, better educated, much more disciplined and basically a more mature human being. She was also blonde, pretty, athletic and fun, so all was good.

As we dated in college, she always did her best to help me keep a rudder in the water and more or less on task. Pat was majoring in special education and was passionate about a teaching career of working with children with special needs. I was more passionate about our next intramural football or basketball game, the upcoming weekend activities and the efforts to scrape up $20 for our upcoming date. Fortunately, with steady doses of Pat's "encouragement," I didn't completely screw up my college education.

When Pat graduated in 1981...I did not. I was still 20 hours short of earning my degree in business management. That summer I took a job as a petroleum landman-trainee in Oklahoma City. My plan was to work over the summer and come back to Norman in the fall to finish my degree—either in one long, butt-kicking grind of a semester or one easy, last-hoorah year of partying. Unfortunately, the greed of a paycheck got in the way of this decision. At the end of that summer, my boss offered me a full-time job. "You don't need that college degree," he said. "I don't even have a degree. Plus, you can always go back later and get it."

Bad advice, which I took. I figured I could go to school at night and finish my degree in one year, anyway—no big deal. But it was, in fact, a big deal because OU didn't offer the classes at night that I needed, and I was really tired of school at that point. I resigned myself to being a working man—a degreeless working man.

But when Pat and I got married the following June, I miraculously grew up. I enrolled at a more night-class-friendly college in Edmond, kept working full-time as a landman, and finally graduated a year and a half later.

We were living the life—college graduates, newlyweds, lots of fun friends, not much money, but all was good. We joined a church, got a dog, bought a house, had a baby—hitting all the stops on the roadmap of life. All was good…or so we thought.

What happened during April through July of 1986 was definitely not on our so-called "roadmap" to our life.

3

Acceptance

From April through July 1986, I was definitely riding the roller coaster of life. Each week was filled with medical appointments, diagnostic tests with no answers, good days, not-so good days, and lots of waiting—waiting for this blindness to decide what it was going to do with me. Yes, the unknown was scary, but I honestly felt like this was a challenge I'd figure out how to manage. One of the doctors along the way said, "It's going to take some guts." I believe he was just thinking this to himself, but the words came out of his mouth. Well, guts I have; brains, sometimes not so much.

As the weeks went by, I began to feel that the chances of regaining my sight were decreasing—that maybe this was not just a temporary thing. If I had noticed even the slightest improvement, then I would have felt some optimism. But I knew that with no improvement to the damaged optic nerve tissue, time was not on my side.

Slowly it was sinking in that I was facing a future completely unimaginable just a few months earlier. But this realization was accompanied by a firm resolve: "If others can do this, then I can do it—no doubt."

I had a lot of help in forming this attitude.

I grew up Catholic but wasn't really involved other than going to Mass on Sundays. Even then, my attendance was hit-and-miss. Some effort was made by my parents to get us to Mass as a family, but my personal experience was never very deep. For example, I had never even opened a Bible, let alone studied it. When Pat and I married, we attended Mass regularly and made it a part of our life. But reading the Bible? Not a priority.

Soon after I lost my sight, my two sisters bought me a complete set of cassette tapes of the New Testament. Playing these tapes, actually listening to the messages and lessons of Jesus, was something new to me. When I first started listening to the tapes, I immediately felt a comfort and strength I had never experienced by just getting dressed up and walking to church for the obligatory one-hour service. By actually digesting and mentally processing the stories, lessons and explanations told by Jesus and His disciples, my faith was increased, as well as my understanding that I am absolutely and completely known by God. This was not an earth-shattering, lightning strike, sell-my-things-and-follow-some-preacher-on-TV kind of experience, nor was it connected to some secret hope for a miracle to restore my sight. It was simply an understanding of the love of God for His children and my faith and trust in His words. Reading the Bible, sorting through and processing His messages, suddenly gave me the comfort and confidence I needed to meet my challenges. Sure, I had no idea of the various types of challenges and real-life obstacles I'd have to overcome, but growing my faith by processing the many lessons of the Bible seemed to give me a feeling of peace and comfort.

My wife came home one day from a teachers' seminar and told me they had heard a really good motivational speaker named Zig Ziglar. He emphasized handling setbacks by positive thinking and keeping a good attitude. I listened to some of his tapes and bought into his message. The words made good sense to me and helped me to connect the dots in a positive and productive way.

So, part of my daily routine was set: listening to the Bible and then listening to a motivational tape. These couple of hours each day gave me strength and comfort and put fuel in my tank. I didn't know what was around the corner, and I tried not to worry about it. All I knew was that I was gaining confidence in myself.

"If someone else could do this, I could."

After all the medical tests were done, the results examined, the final diagnosis of optic neuritis delivered, learning the nerve tissue was beyond repair, and Dr. Farris issuing the word "permanent," I knew it was time to move on. I was unsure of this new roadmap, and uncertain of the future, but I was determined to find ways to beat this opponent.

Pat was incredibly strong and faithful throughout everything, and we knew we were in this together. We had family and friends calling and coming by to visit and give support in any way they could. I think they saw us accepting this situation as a setback in our lives but nothing we couldn't overcome. We were determined to make the best of it and move forward with our lives, which kept spirits up all around. I had made the choice to be positive rather than negative, because I knew it was a choice. Being negative would not allow me to beat this thing. Again, an attitude reflecting more guts than brains, perhaps, but this was the hand dealt to me and I had things to do.

I remember a phone conversation I had with one of my best friends. He asked me, "Ted, aren't you kind of ticked at God?" My immediate response to him was, "No, I can only get through this with Him. No way could I do it without him. We are in this thing together."

Soon after Pat and I married, well before I lost my sight, she picked up a framed poem titled "Footprints in the Sand." We hung it on a wall in our living room. Little did we know that just a few years later the words would have such profound meaning for us. We repeated the poem over and over, and still find comfort in every word:

Footprints in the Sand*

One night I dreamed a dream.
As I was walking along the beach with my Lord.
Across the dark sky flashed scenes from my life.
For each scene, I noticed two sets of footprints in the sand,
One belonging to me and one to my Lord.
After the last scene of my life flashed before me,
I looked back at the footprints in the sand.
I noticed that at many times along the path of my life,

especially at the very lowest and saddest times,
there was only one set of footprints.
This really troubled me, so I asked the Lord about it.
"Lord, you said once I decided to follow you,
You'd walk with me all the way.
But I noticed that during the saddest and most troublesome times of my life,
there was only one set of footprints.
I don't understand why, when I needed You the most, You would leave me."
He whispered, "My precious child, I love you and will never leave you,
Never, ever, during your trials and testings.
When you saw only one set of footprints,
It was then that I carried you."

*Editor's note: the author of this poem is in dispute.

I've thought some people blamed God for my blindness, like my friend who asked me if I was upset with God. I just don't believe God zaps us and causes the negative things we all experience. If that were the case, then that would make Him some kind of monster, playing little cruel games with us, His earthly puppets. No, bad things just happen. I've always believed it's amazing the human body works as well is it does.

I remember being at church about a year into this "adventure" and saying a prayer before Mass. I suppose I was feeling a little down or overwhelmed that day because the prayer began, in essence, "Hey, God, remember me?" The immediate answer in my head from God was, "Ted, I am your Father, you are my son. I always want the best for you."

What struck me was, yes, he is my Father, and what father doesn't want the best for his child? Fathers can't fight all our battles, but every good father certainly wants the best for his kids, 100% of the time.

Actually, I think God must have a pretty good sense of humor. I mentioned that at the time I lost my sight, we had one child, Matthew, who was just a year old. When the final diagnosis was made and it was time to move on with our lives, I remember telling Pat, "Well, no more kids. I know what

Matt looks like, and I'll be able to visualize him as he grows up." Being the good Catholics we are, we used natural family planning as our "birth control" to prevent any more kids because I was convinced I just couldn't handle not knowing what any of my children looked like. Well, here's how that went: Luke was born on July 4, 1988, Samuel in September 1991, Daniel in February 1993, and Anna in June 1995. So much for planning around things "I just couldn't handle." God truly knows best.

And, as the old saying goes, He works in mysterious ways, too.

A couple of months into losing my sight, my dad got a call from one of my high school friends back in Tulsa. He informed my parents that he and a few others had started a fund on my behalf. The word was out about my condition, and donations were being mailed directly to a bank account in Tulsa. Now, the Italian in me is usually too proud to take any handouts, but when Dad informed me of this, I was grateful and very touched. Our health insurance was pretty good, but didn't cover all of our medical expenses, and with our limited income at that time, we were stretching things along the best we could. This money would be used to help Pat and me with medical bills, household expenses and anything else we needed.

When all was said and done, these donations totaled close to $8,000—a generous amount of money that certainly took the edge off the financial strain we were feeling. But the far greater effect of this generosity was the strength we gained in knowing that distant friends were silently thinking of us and doing what they could to make a bad thing a little better.

Now that I knew blindness was a part of my life, it was time to learn to be a blind person and get on with things.

Does an operator's manual exist?

4

The Rookie

Ok, so now it's time to learn the tricks of the trade. Where to start? Perhaps the tap, tap, tap of that white cane, a cool-looking German Shepherd guide dog, or maybe learning to play the piano.

Well, due to lack of musical talent, the piano thing was surely out. Contrary to popular belief, being blind doesn't magically make one musically gifted. The cane thing, however, seemed important for mobility and, maybe most important, safety.

I contacted the State of Oklahoma Visual Services office and told them of my situation: "I've suddenly lost my sight and you have a rookie on your hands." I was informed that they could get me started on some basics, but added that I would need to enroll at an independent living skills rehabilitation center.

Oklahoma does not have such a training facility, but a neighboring state did. However, the waiting list was six months. So, I signed up to begin training in February 1987. I was told to plan on being at the facility for three to six months, possibly longer, depending on my progression with "skills and capabilities."

The primary training offered by our state was focused on cane technique, mobility and braille lessons. I began my training with lessons at home once or twice a week, getting familiar with a cane and practicing orientation skills around my neighborhood. Then I graduated to downtown, on city buses, in shopping malls and any other seemingly torturous situation the instructor wanted me to learn on that particular day. Even though I wasn't working or spending much time traveling solo out of the house, it was important to get up to speed on mobility and orientation skills. The brain quickly learns to process the tactical recognition of hard obstacles, surface changes from hard to soft, slight elevation changes, steps up and down, mid-height tree or bush branches, etc. Head-level, overhanging obstacles still proved a problem, but I learned that a good, experienced cane traveler is able to gain perception when approaching various potential perils. Let's just say I was an average cane user, so I experienced my share of battle scars.

Part of good orientation is knowing where you are at all times, know-ing the route to take you where you are going, traveling solo and arriving in one piece. No, being blind does not give you Superman-like hearing, either, but you do depend on many sounds that sighted people typically pay little attention to, such as parallel or perpendicular traffic, other footsteps, running water, distant trains, buses and irritated dogs. So, it may seem like our hearing is stronger or better, but really it's only because our mind's eye (ear) pays closer attention to helpful sounds. My training also included learning the impor-tance of being oriented to one-way streets, traffic lights versus stop signs, a specific fountain located at a certain point, and other details in my environ-ment. You quickly learn which restaurants or shops normally play music heard from the street, alleys with smelly dumpsters, the pigeons' favorite church rooftops, and other sensory-friendly landmarks.

I was always fairly athletic, so I figured I'd glide along like no big deal. Overall, the early stages of learning cane mobility seemed smooth enough, but I'm sure I didn't look nearly as accomplished as I thought I looked—probably stiff and a bit klutzy. One thing I had going for me: I'm about 6'4" and weigh about 225 pounds, so I usually came out okay with any accidental person-to-person collisions along the way.

I felt I'd eventually want a guide dog, but I learned that before one can be ready to apply for one, a person must have good orientation skills, which makes good sense. I had plenty of work to do with all things related to travel-ing with a cane, so the guide dog idea would be down the road.

The cane and mobility training moved along pretty well, but learn-ing braille was a different story. I was told that it was much easier to learn this sensory language as a child. Why? For one thing, a child's fingertips are smooth and sensitive, and a kid's brain can just process the information easier. As adults, our fingertips are tougher, don't have the sensitivity to easily identify the braille letter or word, and it takes our brains longer to process this new language—or so the kind, patient instructor told me. But this did make sense, at least as far as the tougher fingertips. For me, it was just slower for my fingers to pick up on the bumpy dots.

Basically, think of braille as a domino, with the six dots showing where one or more of the raised braille dots can be located. Various arrangements of the different dots represent a letter, and sometimes a single letter can represent an entire word, somewhat like shorthand. Some people can read braille as quickly as they can run their index finger over the letters and words. These people are very impressive. As for me, I felt like I was all thumbs. Braille was going to be quite the challenge. I decided that I'd learn it the best I could and move on from there.

Each week I continued to work on my cane and braille skills, trying to be patient as I waited for my stay at the independent living skills center. During this time, I became aware of the many tools and assorted gadgets to help the blind: talking clocks and calculators, small Dictaphone tape recorders for taking verbal notes, and other improvised tools. One Saturday afternoon, two ladies from the Pi Beta Phi alumni club of Pat's OU sorority came by the house and gave me a braille wristwatch. I didn't even know there was such a thing. The crystal was on a small hinge and could be popped up by using your thumbnail, enabling me to feel the hour and minute hands to tell the time. It was very cool and I was touched by the gift. It was another example of distant friends reaching out to us.

When late August came around, it was time for Pat to get geared up to go back to her teaching job. We had Matt lined up to go back to the same full-time childcare as the previous year, but I proposed an idea: Why not let me keep him two days a week at home? We could save a little money on childcare and I could spend some extra time bonding with my son. What could possibly go wrong?

Pat consented, and not much went all that wrong, actually. Yes, there was the 250-count package of baby wipes getting strewn around Matt's room in the time it took me to let the dog back in the house, and maybe a little smudge of apple sauce here and there. I think I got pretty good at changing a diaper, though. To me, things were pretty clean if there was no lingering smell.

But there was that one trip to the emergency room.

I was in the backyard with Matt and must have become distracted or maybe I was just letting him run around, chasing the dog. The yard was fenced, so no way for a kid to escape. Then I heard a screech. I got to Matt and found he had climbed the four-foot-high fence and cut his hand on the top spike.

Tears, blood and a call to the neighbor. "You'd better call Pat," said the neighbor. "This looks like a trip to the ER." Pat scrambled home from school and off we went for our first child's first set of stitches. "It could've happened to anybody," we reasoned.

Again, I tried to look at the positive side of everything. I remember thinking, "How many dads get to bond with their one-year-old like this?" Each week, Matt and I had two full days of quality time to build with blocks, wrestle with stuffed animals and enjoy a nap together. Pat picked up several children's books that came with follow-along audio tapes—animated voices that read the words of the story. Each tape included an audible tone notifying the user when to turn the page, so it was a perfect fit for our situation.

One night our good friends, Craig and Nancy Ferguson, invited us over for dinner. We wanted a relaxing, adult evening, so we secured a babysitter and off we went. After dinner, and a couple of beers, Craig looked at me and said, "Come on, let's take the wives dancing."

"Excuse me?"

"Come on, Ted, you'll figure it out. You always thought you were a good dancer, anyway."

This was a conspiracy. Pat loves to dance. Whenever she hears dance music with a little bump in it, she develops a twitch or bodily tick and her hips and shoulders start doing their thing. I was outvoted.

I quickly recognized that dancing is very visual. I think a lot of the real enjoyment of dancing is watching and smiling at your partner, but this was not about me—her hips were on the go, so I had another life lesson to learn. We held hands, which helped with mobility and orientation, and let the music do its job—a little swing here, a little hip bump there, elbows in and all surrounding dancers beware. Hopefully, my hip bumps landed on the right hips. Pat got very good at maneuvering us around the dance floor, and this experience taught us another way to maneuver through one of many new life lessons.

About a month after Pat returned to teaching, she walked in one day, a little teary-eyed, and said, "Those teachers are such good people. They're just so nice." That day, unbeknownst to Pat, the teachers had passed a hat around the break room over lunch and taken donations for us. They had tossed in over $300. We all know teachers are not well paid, so this gesture had even greater impact on us. "Don't spend this money on bills," they instructed Pat. "Go have some fun."

The OU-Texas football game in Dallas was a few weeks away, so "have fun" we did. We made plans to take the trip. We knew several friends who were already planning on going for the weekend, so we joined them. It was a great break and a good chance to visit and catch up with some college friends we hadn't seen in several years. Our dancing friends, Craig and Nancy, insisted we stay in their room and all was set. In an adjoining room would be another couple, also longtime friends. I think they spread the word Pat and I were "in" for the weekend and the party was on, just like old times.

When the football season arrived that fall, I immediately realized the game action described by the commentators was very limited to anyone who can't actually see what's happening on TV. These guys understandably assume that everyone is watching the action on the screen, so very little of value (to me) is added by their commentary. Because of this, I began to rely on a radio broadcast to follow the actual action. Most play-by-play radio announcers are very impressive; they understand that the listener is depending on them to describe the game with such verbal details as yard lines, uniform colors, substitutions, formations, holes created by good blocking, quarterbacks in trouble, ranting coaches, etc. Rarely do you hear these colorful, graphic details from a TV commentator. I very rarely missed the radio coverage of my beloved Oklahoma Sooners, via small Walkman headphones plugged into my ears. At times this is a little awkward at an occasional watch party, with all others sitting around watching the game unfold on TV while I'm tuned into my radio. But if it was a Sooner football or basketball game, like most Sooner fans I hung on every play.

A month or so later, I got a phone call from a good friend of mine, David Reeves. "Brian, Tony and I want to get you out of the house and give Pat a break," said David. "We'll pick you up next Saturday and go to Kansas City for a steak dinner and a Chiefs football game. What do you think?"

It sounded great—a fun weekend with three old buddies. The four of us did everything together in high school, and two of us attended OU together. I looked forward to lots of old stories, rehashing those types of high school and college tales that just won't die. They picked me up that Saturday morning and we were off to KC.

We started getting hungry around lunch time and asked David, our driver, to stop somewhere for a quick lunch. "No way, we're not eating," he snorted. "We've got a big KC steak dinner waiting on us for dinner and we need to be good and hungry. It'll just taste that much better."

I really don't like to skip meals. Sometimes I even get a little shaky, so I asked, "OK, but how about just a little snack to hold us over?"

He did pull over at the next store and ran inside. He returned with no snacks—only beer. "Man, that steak is going to taste great," Dave reminded us.

We checked into our hotel and walked over to the Golden Ox Steakhouse, a Kansas City steak institution. We were starving and the smell was awesome. We arrived at about 6:00 and, of course, there was an hour wait. Our ring-leader, Big Dave, downplayed this delay. "That's good news. Just think how hungry we'll really be in an hour," he said.

So, we decided to walk back to the hotel lobby to wait because we had noticed earlier that the hotel offered complimentary drinks and hors d'oeuvres. We did get a drink, but Dave, of course, nixed even the thought of us splitting an order of potato skins. "It might ruin our dinner," he said. At this point, we hadn't eaten in about 12 hours.

We returned to the restaurant, the smell still awesome, and were seated. We were starving and may have even thanked Dave for making us hold out for this coveted moment. When the steaks were brought to the table, all was right in the world—or so I thought. Suddenly, the day caught up with me and I started feeling a little shaky.

"Hey, Brian, can you help me to the bathroom or outside for a little fresh air?" I asked. We stood up, I took Brian's elbow, walked about four steps and down I went. I felt faint, but didn't completely pass out. I just felt incredibly weak. As I lay there on the floor, I heard Brian actually say, "Is there a doctor in the house?!"

The next thing I heard was a voice saying, "I'm a doctor, what's wrong?"

"He's blind, you know, optic neuritis," Brian explained. Probably not the diagnosis the doctor was looking for at that moment. Not that he listened anyway. Our hero/doctor, who had a big cigar in his mouth, got in my face and held up three fingers. "How many fingers?" he asked the blind man. Brian told me later that he held up his "one" finger in this doctor's face.

We finished our dinner, went to see the Raiders beat our Chiefs the next day, and returned home under an oath of silence.

As the cane and braille skills moved along, I figured out other ways to improvise daily activities to be as functional and normal as possible, like keeping socks matched by using safety pins, putting certain items in the same place in the fridge, using tactical marks on some appliances, and other simple, basic stuff. I thought working out would be a good stress reliever, so I held on to the baby seat on the back of Pat's bike and we'd go for a run. It probably looked weird, but doing things a little differently was something I needed to accept. We continued to learn to do such things and embrace our new way of life.

During these initial six or eight months of experiencing my blindness and this new life, I didn't really feel a sense of urgency. It was more a sense of persistence, tolerance, motivation, and dealing with a very unique challenge that relatively few others would experience. I accepted that it was real, it was here, and it was me. I had no choice in the matter. I knew it was a new life, as well as a journey that I would take on and learn to manage.

I was nervously looking forward to my full-time rehab stay in February. I could learn to work around many basic living skills through common sense and trial and error, but I knew I needed to learn many other "tricks of the trade" from rehabilitation professionals at an in-house, full-time learning environment.

5

Rehab Me

As the calendar grew closer to my rehab trip in February, I took a mental inventory of my situation.

The physical part of me seemed pretty good. I was in decent shape and healthy. I've always had a big appetite and, thankfully, a good metabolism. Over the previous ten months, I hadn't been as active with my old favorites such as weekly adult pick-up basketball games at church, summer company softball league and longer runs, so with my big-boy appetite and habit of eating everything and anything I wanted, I knew I'd better watch it. But I felt fortunate I was able to easily stay in shape.

My mental and emotional inventory was still in pretty good shape, as well. Of course, some days were frustrating and the unknown continued to be a little worrisome, but I stayed positive and maintained a productive, can-do attitude. I continued to fuel my tank with my daily routine of motivational tapes and Bible readings. Again, I had a choice to stay positive each day. Maybe it's the competitive nature in me, but I knew the only way to enjoy the parts of this different life was to move forward with what I had, and not feel defeated by what I had lost. I don't want to minimize the frustration and limits we as blind go through; it takes constant effort and some good, helpful people along the way. But I knew many things were achievable and I was determined to make things as normal as possible.

Adding to my determination was the fact that Pat and I had a child to raise, and I knew children learn and develop their attitudes from watching and being around their parents and home environment. I felt that if I used this setback as an excuse to not be productive and successful, then Matt would learn to use an excuse when things get tough. It's a cliché, I know, but one lesson we all teach our kids is: "If you get thrown off your horse, get back on." Does this not apply to adults as well? I knew that, over time, Matt would be watching and learning, so my attitude would be a reflection of my character. I also knew I had a mountain to climb and you can only accomplish big challenges by remaining positive.

When February arrived, I was ready to go. I wasn't looking forward to being out of state and away from my family for several months, but I was ready to move this project on to the next learning stage. Our plan was for me to fly home once a month, provided we could continue to stretch the finances. The thought of a monthly visit was encouraging and would make being away for an extended time more tolerable. Pat and I knew this in-house, intense training was a necessary part of my learning to be the best I could be, so not going was not an option. I knew I'd learn to do things better and discover new ways of doing more things to help me be better equipped to be as independent as possible. I didn't know what lay ahead of me in the next few months, let alone the next few years, but it was time to prepare for it.

On the first Saturday of February 1987, Pat, Matt and I loaded into our car and made the four-hour drive out of state to the independent learning skills rehab center. It was a feeling of good and bad—good that I was going to learn things, bad in the form of the unknown and being away from my family and friends. I guess it was a lot like a kid being sent off to boarding school.

We pulled up to the facility late that afternoon. I got checked in and we were given a tour of the facility. To be quite honest, the environment was a real downer. Pat and I both felt this way. It had an institutional feel to it. Pat noticed many students just hanging around, looking unmotivated and unenergetic. To be fair, it was a Saturday afternoon so it may have been a slow time, but the overall mood just seemed depressing.

We were going to stay the night in a hotel, go to church in the morning, and then Pat and Matt would hit the road back to Oklahoma City while I got ready for Monday morning training. But the center had an overnight guest room available, so we opted to not get a hotel and stay at the center.

This may or may not have been such a good idea. The more Pat was around the "institution," the more upset she got about the surroundings. She is a strong, ambitious, optimistic person, so this type of negative feeling is foreign to both of us. As she slowly got more upset, I became upset. Even two-year-old Matt started to cry, and I remember thinking, "Even he senses that something just doesn't feel right." I think the combination of this environment, the pending extended stay and reality of this lifelong road hit us in an unexpected way, without warning. The thought of my being away from home and in this facility for several months hit us between the eyes, and it was discomforting.

Had we not grasped the reality of my situation? Did we underestimate the endless challenges and restrictions of what it was really like to be blind—or being married to someone blind—in the real world? Maybe being in our comfortable home environment, surrounded by the love and support of our family and friends, put us in a type of la-la land, and we were somehow in denial of the magnitude of losing my sight.

My first few days at the rehab facility were sobering and very real, but I was more determined than ever to learn, stay motivated and retain a positive outlook. I was not naïve; I understood things would always be difficult. For example, I learned that the unemployment rate for the blind usually hovered around 70%, so the odds against reentering the business world were against me. But I would cross that bridge when I got to it. I knew myself as a person, and I felt somehow things would fall in place if I could continue to take the positive road. The lessons I would learn within this facility would be challenging, as would my life lessons beyond this facility, but it was time to learn from the professionals and prepare myself to be the best I could be.

The main focus of the school was to get each student to be proficient primarily in cane travel, braille and typing. With the most intense training focused on these three skills, the other training was on general independent living skills such as cooking, sewing, laundry, tying a necktie, handling money and working with basic hand tools. There was also a woodworking shop for both learning a hobby as well as learning a possible trade. Keep in mind, in 1987 the personal computer, Internet, mobile phones and all things related were either in their infant stages or non-existent.

The teachers and guidance counselors were professional and helpful (some of the teachers also were visually impaired). They encouraged the students to work at their own pace, and were patient in dealing with all types of personalities. As you learned their way of each life skill they taught, you would test out of that particular skill and move onto the next class.

The living quarters were basically a dormitory similar to a college setting—a roommate and a bathroom per room, several rooms along long hallways within several wings on three separate floors. One night, sometime after midnight, the fire alarm went off. Picture the scene of a fire alarm going off in a building full of blind people, all heading into the hallways at once. It turned out to be a false alarm, fortunately, so it was really kind of funny—at least to me. Remember, I'm 6'4" and 225 pounds, so I usually come out OK on the bodily "fender benders."

I was amazed at how smooth and fluid some of these guys maneuvered around the halls and classrooms with their canes. Some blind have limited vision, and I think having even the smallest amount of vision would be helpful in moving around. But some guys at the center could sneak up without a sound and be standing right next to you. I knew I'd never be one of those guys. As my wife frequently says: "You're lumbering."

As the days rolled on, I got to know some of these guys fairly well. We had our share of fun and I picked up on various ways of getting around. The bottom line in most situations is that what works for some may or may not work for others, and some people are just better with their instincts and intuitions. Of course, most things come smoother and easier with practical experience and time.

As the first weekend approached, some of the guys who had been around for some time started talking about a bar a couple of blocks down the road. They invited me to go have a beer. You could not have alcohol on the facility grounds, but you could go off campus to "relax," so I assumed we'd be fine. It sounded fun and a beer might just hit the spot—unless this was a joke on the new guy, a snipe hunt or some sort of initiation to the club. The bar did exist, however, so it was not a joke, but I guess it *was* a type of initiation of drinking with my blind brethren.

So, we enjoyed our little getaway and then, "Uh-oh…," it was time to go. I only had a couple of beers, but I knew getting back to the center was definitely going to be an adventure. By depending on a cane for traveling, the situation could be referred to as a sort of "drinking and driving." Of course, some of the guys would slur, "I'm in good shape; here, hold onto my elbow." Well, nothing like a couple of guys forgetting proper, formal cane technique, wildly swinging canes all over the place and driving themselves into a ditch. I figured the next weekend it would be much smarter—and safer—to bring (sneak) a six-pack back to the dorm room and enjoy a quiet evening in our room with a couple of the guys. Something told me sneaking the beer into our room would be easy, as our dorm monitor was also blind.

I noticed over that first week there was a student who always had a heavy key ring full of keys on his belt. Why in the world did he need all of those keys? The word got out that he wore them to make noise so some blind person wouldn't run into him. I guess he thought he was special and needed to put himself in some sort of protective bubble. Well, I thought this was arrogant on his part and it kind of rubbed me wrong, so one day, for one of the few times in my life, I played the "Sorry, I'm blind" card…and "accidentally" T-boned him. It felt pretty good.

After the second week, I noticed some of the guys were taking time off during the day and didn't have a full class schedule. Some were spending a lot of time in the wood shop or leisurely playing braille cards or backgammon during the day. The school really didn't push anyone; you just basically moved at your own pace. Maybe these guys were single (or wished they were) or just weren't real motivated to get home. Maybe they were just relaxing and enjoying time with others, or a combination of these factors, but I wanted to get this stage of my life done and move on. I was getting through the basic classes fairly quickly, so I approached the counselor and posed this question: If I continued to test out of the basics, would there be a chance I could get back home sooner rather than later? She indicated I could probably go home as soon as I got through all the basics, and then I could continue to work on cane, mobility and braille out of my house, using the services provided by the State of Oklahoma.

This was all I needed to hear. My cane and mobility skills were not bad. My braille was bad and probably would never be very good, so that would be a long-term project anyway. If I could go home within a couple of weeks rather than a couple of months, I'd definitely be more motivated than ever.

Again, I don't want to minimize or simplify the challenges of functioning as a blind person or the valuable lessons taught at this rehab center. I'm not trying to criticize or question another's effort, abilities or daily challenges, but I felt I had such good support with friends and family that it was probably easier for me than for most to stay hopeful and positive in what I was dealing with.

At the end of the third week, it looked very likely I'd be done in one more week, so the counselors and I made sure to stay on track, check things off the list and make preparation for me to move on. One of the discussions we had concerned the use of a guide dog instead of a cane. This is obviously a personal choice and there are pros and cons. Anyone who wants to use a guide dog must have acceptable mobility and orientation skills, and the guide dog counselor would make this determination during an in-home interview as a part of the application process. The rehab center has nothing to do with the guide dog school other than providing some information on guide dog schools around the country.

I told my counselor that I had been thinking for several months about utilizing a guide dog instead of a cane. He recommended the two oldest and largest guide dog schools in the country. "They're very good, well established and have good reputations," he said. "One is in Morristown, New Jersey, and the other is in Northern California, in San Rafael, across the bay from San Francisco."

"New Jersey or California?"

"Yes."

Nothing against Jersey, but to me this was a very, very easy decision. I like the New York area, but it's not Northern California.

"Please pick up the phone and call the place in San Rafael and get me on the list," I impatiently said. He did as I requested and learned that there was a three-month waiting list. May was as soon as I could get in.

"I'll take it!"

At the end of the fourth week, I was good to go. I had become familiar with many things and been trained on how to deal with certain daily skills and situations. I knew I had lots of things to practice, but I felt confident and comfortable enough to move on from the in-house rehab, pack my bags and get home to Oklahoma City for "re-entry."

Little did I know that I was just a couple of short weeks away from a phone call that would change my life.

6

Game Changer

Getting back to my routine in Oklahoma City was a great feeling. I felt true relief that the out-of-state rehab experience was behind me. Not only did I get exposed to some life situations and introduced to skills and tools to help me deal with daily issues, I also learned how to troubleshoot in an efficient way and gained confidence in my problem-solving abilities. That one month of rehab, along with my now one year of day-to-day experience, allowed me to stay positive and confident that I could improvise through many potential obstacles.

When reviewing and evaluating where I was at that time, I remember thinking, "Yes, this will always be challenging and I'll have to learn to deal with many situations. With time comes experience, and with experience comes improvement, which leads to attacking and obtaining goals and objectives." I only had a small amount of blind experience during that first year, and I had a mountain of life to experience before meeting the many obstacles ahead. Nobody starts a new and uncharted journey with experience, or feels qualified to succeed or meet all objectives. Experience leads to growth.

I continued to receive weekly training in mobility, orientation and braille lessons from the State of Oklahoma rehabilitation services. It was now practice, practice, practice. I was scheduled to travel to California in May, just two short months away. I was excited to learn to use a guide dog, as I had heard traveling with a dog usually makes the user more independent, more efficient and able to walk at a quicker pace. However, the thought of being dropped off for a month in another dreary, institutional-type facility was nothing to be excited about. But the guide dog would be another useful tool, so we'd make the best of it.

I'd been home from rehab about a week when the phone rang one evening. It was Pat's cousin from Tulsa, Jim Langdon. Jim is a great guy and we'd become good friends from the time I started dating Pat back in college. He asked about the next time we'd be in Tulsa. It just so happened that we had plans to go to Tulsa the following weekend to visit my mom. Jim said he and his wife, Juley Roffers, wanted to invite Pat and me over for dinner and introduce me to a guy named Robert Hutton, whose family knew Pat's family from their roots in Henryetta. I knew Robert's older brother, Richard, who was good friends with Pat's parents. We'd stop by and visit Richard and his family whenever we spent time in Henryetta, but I'd never met Robert.

Two weeks later we were at the Langdon's, having dinner with Robert and his wife, Dana. All were curious about my out-of-state rehab stay and how things had been going over the past several months. Robert said he had kept up with me through Jim and Richard. He then told me that he and some partners had bought a small oil and gas company in Tulsa a couple of years earlier. They were growing the base business and had also started an affiliated natural gas marketing company.

"Ted," said Robert, "I like your background as a landman and I like your attitude, so I'd like to offer you a job."

"Offer me a job?"

"You bet. I've heard there is some type of talking computer equipment and scanners and who-knows-what other kinds of useful technology for the blind out there. We can get you all set up and make it happen. What do you think?"

"Robert, I don't know what to say. This is quite a surprise. Thank you."

The offer came out of the blue. Obviously, it seemed like a potential game-changer and an absolute answer to prayer.

Robert added, "You've had a crappy hand dealt to you and you need a break, so this is your break. You deserve it."

Pat and I had no idea this was planned at this dinner. Pat and Robert knew each other from the family's friendship. It was an unforeseen gift.

"You and Pat go home and talk about it and let me know if this is something you'd consider," said Robert.

"There is nothing to think about—I'm in," I said with immense gratitude.

"OK, great. Please check with your state visual services counselor on what type of computer equipment you'll need, and then come by the office in the next couple of weeks and we'll get it ordered. It will be here waiting on you when you get back from guide dog school. Can you start July 1st?"

When I returned to my mom's house after dinner, we announced this "news from heaven" and a true family hug was the only appropriate thing to do. I know this gave my mother great relief, as she was under constant worry over me. The real cherry on top for Mom was that we'd be moving to Tulsa. As Pat, Matt and I drove back to Oklahoma City the next day, we could not have asked for a better gift. It was unbelievable, a true miracle for us. All seemed good.

As we celebrated this amazing gift, the one thing we hadn't thought of was the necessity of suddenly having to sell our house. At the time, the housing market in Oklahoma City was ugly. The price of oil had not recovered from the low of $9 per barrel over the past year. We loved our house. It was very nice, not too big or too small, and in an established neighborhood. Of course, I was starting my new job July 1st, with or without selling this house, so Pat and I would find a way to make everything happen. I was going to be in California the entire month of May, and I hated the idea of Pat dealing with trying to sell our house alone.

It turns out that our blessing was not restricted to my getting a new job, as God decided to put a bow on it. Within 30 days of putting our house on the market, we received a contract—one week before leaving for California. Once again, my thoughts returned to how we were surrounded by amazing friends and family and how so many things just seemed to fall in place. Sure, the blindness was a constant challenge, and I knew it would be with me forever, but I had many things for which to be thankful. I had a loving, determined wife, a healthy, happy child, and so many good people in what seemed like a growing community of good friends. It made my life much easier to stay motivated and move forward on a positive track.

After we received the great news of the job, our good friends, Tim and Pam Boyle, invited us over for dinner to celebrate. The four of us had gone to college together, so we knew each other very well. Tim and Pam had two little girls and we had Matt, so it was an evening of just hanging out, with lots of diapers, toys and good kid time. After dinner, Pam decided to perm Pat's hair in the kitchen. I went into the kitchen a little later to get something to drink and noticed that both girls were leaning over the sink, messing with Pat's hair. Feeling a little chipper, I gave Pat's hiney a little scratch—only it wasn't Pat's hiney. Wrong rump! Pam immediately looked at Pat with a startled face. After the initial embarrassment, we all enjoyed a good laugh. That story, and laugh, was relived for weeks. It was an innocent, and poorly executed, gesture on my part, but another lesson learned.

Now that we had manna from heaven in the form of a job in Tulsa, we had an agenda and a true path to our future. Pat loved her teaching job in Oklahoma City, but my job opportunity in Tulsa was such a gift. Our life plan would now be focused on my one-month training at guide dog school in May, packing, closing on our house in June and moving to Tulsa, where Pat would look for a teaching position.

Our neighbors in Oklahoma City were sad to see us leave, but they were all happy, and proud, that we'd landed on our feet with a new opportunity in Tulsa. These special friends had been there from the initial days of my losing my sight. They had provided meals, spontaneous yard work, babysitting and anything else they could think of doing to help us out—more examples of the many wonderful, positive people surrounding us.

7

More Than Man's Best Friend

As May approached and I was finalizing my trip to guide dog school in California, we had another visit from two women of the Pi Phi alumni club. I thoroughly appreciated the braille watch they had given me soon after I lost my sight, and this surprise visit gave me another chance to thank them. The alumni club members had caught wind that I was going to California for guide dog school and had come by with another gift.

"Pat," said Mary, "the area outside of San Francisco where this school is located is beautiful, so you need to go with Ted for a little mini-vacation. You guys could go a few days before Ted needs to check into the school and enjoy the city. We want to send you. We'll take care of your plane ticket and the hotel. My husband and I have stayed at the Sir Francis Drake Hotel in San Francisco and loved it, so we suggest you guys stay there. Is that okay with you?"

"Wow!"

So, so many thoughtful, caring and supportive people.

The guide dog school was in San Rafael, just across the bay from San Francisco. Neither of us had ever been to that area of the country, and the thought of my being away for another month of training and rehab made the gift of this trip that much more special.

The three-day mini-vacation in that "beautiful city by the bay" was great. The two of us being together in an incredible, historic place, along with the comfort of having my job on the horizon, helped minimize my dread of whatever type of facility I was about to encounter.

With our mini-vacation over, the plan was for us to rent a car on that Sunday morning, have Pat drive me to the school and get me checked in and settled, then drive herself to the airport for the flight home. Throughout the 30-minute drive to the school from San Francisco, not much was said, mainly due to what we experienced upon arriving at the independent learning rehab facility just a couple of months before. So, here we were headed to another one of those training experiences. "Deal with it and move on" was my attitude.

Our worries could not have been more unfounded. As Pat turned through the gate of the campus, she immediately felt uplifted. "Oh, this is beautiful!" she commented. We drove up the winding entrance road to the main administration building of Guide Dogs For The Blind, Inc., and parked. The school is located on a ten-acre campus with rolling hills in the middle of Marin County, just outside of San Rafael. It was a beautiful, sunny, late morning in May. Pat described the scene: people and dogs all around, walking, working, laughing and seeming happy and content to be doing what they were doing. She saw students outside enjoying the sun and surroundings, dog trainers working with dogs and joking with passersby, energetic volunteers helping in the kennel, and the staff just reflecting California cool. Within five minutes of arriving, we both knew this facility would be night and day compared to my past extended, in-house training experience. It could have been the weather, the open and comfortable surroundings, the clean buildings situated around the campus, the kicked-back attitude of both staff and students or just the energy of the environment, but we immediately sensed this was a very positive and exciting place. Other than being away from the wife and kid, this month looked like a good one on the front end.

My roommate was a minister from a small town outside of Tulsa. The school obviously tried to match roommates with people with similar backgrounds or areas of the country. This guy had lost his sight in the Vietnam War about 13 or 14 years prior and had just now decided to get his first guide dog. He was a great guy with a great attitude, and it was nice to have some common ground, being from Oklahoma. It was also refreshing to be around someone who had dealt positively with losing his sight, was married with a family, had a career and possessed a pleasant, fun personality.

One of my classmates, Adelle Moeller, lived about one hour away and her husband, Mike, was coming to visit the next Sunday so they could attend church together in San Rafael. The school offered volunteers each Sunday to take anyone to their church of choice, so I had planned on going to the local Catholic church with a volunteer. But Adelle insisted I go with her and her husband to the Catholic church, so I did.

On the way back from Mass, Mike asked, "Ted, you ever play golf?"

"Oh, I played a little before I lost my sight, but not very well," I said.

"I've got some clubs in the trunk. Do you want to check with the school and see if you can go with me to the driving range and hit a few balls?"

I thought it sounded like a fun idea. Sundays were slow at school; we only had one or two short meetings and only a little work with the dogs (both dog and student needed a little mental rest after a busy six-day work week). So, we did go out and hit a few balls and I wasn't too bad—probably about the same as prior to losing my sight. But I kept this information to myself.

All first-time guide dog users must go through a 30-day training program. To handle and care for a guide dog, there are many rules, restrictions and guidelines to learn and abide by. It was critical to understand the importance of your training, the do's and don'ts of using the dog, especially the consistency both user and dog will need to live by. Even though these dog trainers are pleasant and easygoing by nature, they are professionals and very good at what they do. More important, they understand the seriousness, and danger, of a dog and user not traveling well together. If a guide dog is inconsistent or lazy, and a blind person hasn't learned to properly handle and trust the dog one hundred percent, then both dog and user can find themselves in a potentially dangerous situation.

Many blind are very comfortable and confident with using canes, which I certainly understand. So, when a blind person decides to make the move to using a guide dog, it's a big decision. It's very much a leap of faith to put away the comforts of a cane and learn to trust an animal. This is a true commitment.

Part of the application process for being admitted to a guide dog school is an in-house interview by someone from the school. This interview takes place in the applicant's home well before being enrolled in the school. The purpose is to not only ensure that the person has considered all aspects of utilizing a guide dog, but also to assess the person's orientation and mobility skills, as well as his/her long-term commitment to putting away the cane and trusting the dog. I was new to this blind world, did not grow up traveling with a cane, so I was certainly not attached to the idea of relying on a cane for maneuvering through obstacles. I knew there would be pros and cons of using a dog, but I always felt using a guide dog was the way to go for me. I read somewhere that under ten percent of blind people use a guide dog. Did this majority know something I didn't? I didn't know for sure, but I did know I had much to learn at this school.

There were about 25 students in my class. Most were from the West Coast, but there were the two Okies and several from Colorado, Chicago and Boston. It was about half men and women, a few in their 20s but the majority in their 30s and 40s. They came from all backgrounds and situations, some newly blind and some blind for many years. It seemed to be an educated, well-versed and diverse group of outgoing, energetic people.

There was also a class of about ten students who had come back to get their second, third or fourth guide dog. Once you've gone through the initial month-long training class for your first dog, you only need two weeks of retraining for your subsequent dogs. These two classes were the only students on campus at any one time, so only around 35 students were on site. The "retreads" were veterans, so they roomed in a separate wing and used a separate lounge area for their lessons and lectures, which made sense as they only needed a refresher course and not the cover-to-cover, intense training from the ground floor up.

Each class had two dog trainers who also served as the teachers. There is much to learn and practice prior to working with a dog, so new students don't receive a dog until the fourth day. Also, the trainers needed time to learn about the students' walking pace, true height, personality, home environment (with or without other pets), whether they lived in rural or urban environment, their work situation and other details of their background. All of this information would be used to match the right guide with the right user. The school always worked with a pool of about 40 completely trained guide dogs to pull from and match with the incoming class of students. The dogs were already trained, but the blind users needed a lot of work.

Guide Dogs For The Blind only uses golden retrievers, Labrador retrievers and German shepherds as guides. All dogs are bred at the school and raised in the onsite kennels until they are about 14 weeks old. At that point, each puppy is adopted out to a 4H family and raised under a very structured and organized program monitored by the school. The puppy-raiser, usually a teenager, and the puppy attend monthly meetings, practice specific obedience lessons, attend sporting events, visit shopping malls, high-traffic areas and other situations to get the dog accustomed to what a trained guide dog will experience. When the puppy reaches 14 months old, the dog is returned to the school to begin its formal guide training. This is usually an emotional farewell for the puppy-raiser family members, but also carries a sense of pride for this accomplishment and participation in this important program. Most puppy-raisers are "repeat customers" and will ask to be placed on the list to raise another puppy for the school.

The dogs bred at the school to be guides possess very strong, defined bloodlines. But even through this program—which, in addition to careful raising and strict obedience training, includes six to eight months of highly intensive guide work training—only about 50 percent of the dogs are selected to be guides. Some have potential health issues, some are too large (over 100 pounds is just too much dog for practical use), some show signs of aggression, and others just can't get the training down. This told me that the graduated working guide dogs are the best of the best. The teachers are quick to say the dogs that don't "get it" don't "flunk," but are only "career change" dogs.

On the fourth day, we got our dogs. It is obviously a highly anticipated day. We had gone over the basic, simple training on the how's, why's, do's and don'ts of handling, treating and caring for these dogs, and the overall expectations of owning and using them. The overriding feeling from the students, however, was the excitement and anticipation of traveling in a more independent and efficient manner. Again, cane use is fine for many, and a dog is not for everyone, but if it's your deal, it seemed like the world of maneuvering and traveling was getting ready to open up.

My first dog was a male golden retriever named Gambit. He was a beautiful, 80-pound, easygoing, focused dog that was 100 percent professional. The training had been exceptional and I was more and more impressed every day. We seemed like a perfect match. Of course, this was to be expected as the teachers are very good at what they do when matching a guide with a user. At the moment the dog is placed with the student, they become inseparable, so the bonding period is crucial. These dogs know and love their trainers, so the conversion of loyalty to their new "master" is important and can take several days or weeks. The dog's bed is in the student's room, the student feeds and grooms the dog, and the two spend both class/lecture and leisure time together.

The teachers explained in detail why and how the dogs are trained to do what they do as guides, and it's all very interesting. I continued to be impressed not only with the capabilities of these dogs but also with the teachers as professionals. They were constantly dealing with all types of personalities, emotions, frustrations and assorted challenges experienced by their students, but always remained upbeat, positive and patient, yet firm, in their expectations of both student and dog.

Our days began at 7:00 a.m. with feeding our dogs and then feeding ourselves in the dining hall, followed by lessons and lectures beginning at 8:00. We would then either work the dogs around the campus under teacher supervision or load up on the school bus and go to downtown San Rafael to work in a different setting. Then it was back to campus for lunch, then more afternoon work similar to the morning sessions. The last lecture and/or guide work practice session of the day normally ended around 8:00 or 9:00 p.m., so these were long days for everyone. Two teachers were always present, and they were going strong the whole time. Students got a breather when a teacher worked one-on-one with a student, but the teachers never took a break. It was obvious that they loved what they were doing.

No people food for the dogs—that's one of the rules of training. If a dog gets a little taste of the good stuff, even a small nibble, he'd like it—probably a lot. If you decide to ignore this rule, then what do you think this "professional" guide would be focused on as he's guiding you through a restaurant? He'd be distracted by sniffing the floor for scraps, and the next thing you know you're plowing right into the lady slurping her soup. Not good. These dogs cannot be distracted in restaurants by knowing the taste of people food. A dog's feeding is very regulated, with a specific time in the morning and each evening. At each feeding, you put the food down and he eats, then offer water, then out to relieve. No food or water is left in the bowls throughout the day. Dogs learn to eat the food and drink the water whenever it's offered, because if they don't, they'll learn it won't be offered again for a long period of time. This routine must stay on schedule and be consistent, including the dog's schedule of going out to relieve. Trust me, this is very, very important, or else it can be very, very embarrassing.

I asked my teacher, Bob Wendler, how he got into guide dog work as a profession. He said, "Well, I'll tell ya. I enlisted to join the Army during Vietnam. When I showed up for duty, the enrollment officer asked what area I was interested in, so I told him airplane mechanics. The officer looked at his clipboard and said, 'We're full there. You're in canine. NEXT!' That was that. And the rest is history."

The dogs are trained on very specific things, mainly focused on maneuvering and safety. They are trained to walk down the center of the sidewalk or path, watching for best clearance on either side. They know how to maneuver around any obstacles, including people, along the path without unnecessary stops until they reach the next step up or step down, which is usually the curb at the next perpendicular street. If a dog comes to something unusual blocking the path—such as a downed branch or open manhole cover—and a clear, safe path around this obstacle is not somewhat obvious, then he will stop. At that point, it's up to the user to figure out the reason for the interruption. The user can then work the dog to the left or right to determine if the dog is comfortable and confident enough to go around and pick up the original path. If this is not clear, and the user feels the dog is not confident in working around the obstacle in a safe manner, then it's best to go back and try another route.

The dog understands verbal commands such as "left" and "right" but does not read traffic lights, as some people assume. After the dog has walked to the next intersecting street, he will stop at the down curb and wait for the next command. This is when the user needs to know exactly where he or she is and the direction and route from that point. The user will know it's safe to cross when he hears his parallel traffic surge forward; then it's time to command the dog "forward" across the street until the next curb up, which is where the dog will stop, as trained. At that point, it's another "forward" command to proceed in the same direction or a "halt," then "right" or "left" to travel in that direction.

Part of the training also involves the dog recognizing often-used, familiar doors to offices, restaurants, etc. When the dog recognizes a door, he will slow down and kind of "show" this door to the user. If this is the place, then "Good boy" is offered and the dog will travel directly to that door. If it's not the destination, then he'll hear "No, hop up," which to the dog means to keep traveling down the path.

The dogs are also taught to "intelligently disobey." If a user thinks it's clear to cross the street and gives the "forward" command, but the dog sees something he doesn't like—a bicycle or a construction crew, for example—then he won't go. That's when it's up to the user to trust the dog and figure out why he's uncomfortable with the command.

The first two weeks of training with the dog are good but at times a little shaky, as dog and user get to know and gain confidence in each other. It's understood that some mistakes will be made. Over the first eight or nine days, the teacher travels directly behind the team to assure all is well and going as expected, with only a few suggestions to the user when absolutely necessary. After that time, most work is done independently without a teacher on your heels. The teachers quietly post themselves around an area of town where the students and dogs are traveling, observing and trying to stay ahead of any danger in a student's specific route. Day by day, the dog and user gain confidence and the team becomes smooth and fluid.

Either during the third or early in the fourth week, I was feeling very confident, which is a good thing. But there were times when I actually felt a little cocky, which is a bad thing. For example, one day I thought I'd stop to get an ice cream cone before walking the two blocks back to the student lounge. Big mistake, as one of the teachers posted around the corner witnessed my unsanctioned detour and saw a "learning" opportunity. She quickly stepped in front of me as I left the ice cream store, hoping for a head-on collision, with me smashing ice cream up my nose. Fortunately, Gambit was too good at what he does and stopped just short of this collision.

"Good boy!"

It's a good thing one of us knew what he was doing. But at least I did have a learning experience: no matter what your confidence level is, some things just aren't a good idea.

The school does a great job of trying to expose the dogs and students to all situations and environments. After a couple of weeks of working in San Rafael, we took the bus into San Francisco. We needed to work in a downtown area with all the activities that come with a large city, including busy, high-traffic areas, crowded sidewalks with pedestrians not watching where they're going, homeless people, road construction, sidewalk cafes and everything imaginable, all of which is absolutely necessary to encounter and learn how to navigate properly. The dogs usually do better than the students, so a lot of these training situations are primarily for the student's preparation and confidence. This was important because the time was approaching for user and dog to go home and be on their own.

Unfortunately, two guys in my class didn't make it through training and went home after a couple of weeks. It's normal for a class to lose a student or two. This can be due to the emotions of the student, his inability to trust the dog or himself, a lack of good mobility and orientation skills or some combination of the above. It is the school's priority to be certain that the guide dog and user are completely ready to be on their own in a productive, and safe, manner.

This was a good month for me. Even though I appreciated Gambit just as a good dog, I understood that he was also a tool that I could depend on for tackling the many mobility challenges I'd soon face. I learned a lot and met many good people—not only my fellow students, who along with me were excited and ambitious with our first guide dogs, but also the dog trainers, who I knew were always a phone call away to answer questions or concerns.

Graduation day was a big deal. Hundreds of people attended, including the puppy-raisers. Speeches were given, awards were handed out, and there was an atmosphere of excitement, accomplishment and anticipation of going home to introduce our world to our new four-legged "partners."

Through my attendance at both the independent living facility and the guide dog school, I gained life lessons I never could have imagined before entering these schools. I learned from observing others' and my own practicality. I learned ways of doing basic things differently around the house to contribute to the household chores. And I learned to trust a dog to guide me around the obstacles of life.

I knew I needed to absorb all of these lessons, all of these new ways of doing things, like them or not, if I wanted to continue moving forward in a productive way.

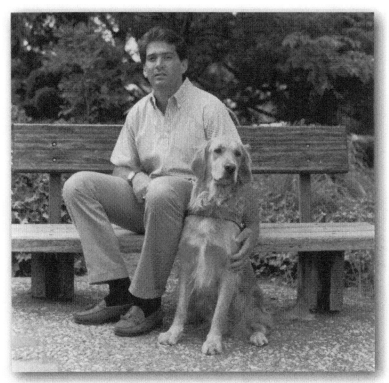

Ted and Gambit, 1st guide dog, May 1987

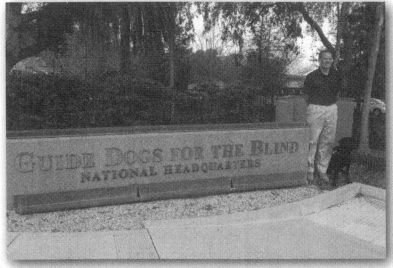

Ted and Kansas, 5th guide dog, February 2017

8

Getting Traction

As Gambit and I were dropped off at the San Francisco airport for our flight home, I had the excitement of going home, confidently traveling more independently and charting new waters with this special guide. But I also had the fear of knowing I was no longer being secretly watched over by the guide dog school teachers. Did I learn everything? Was the dog as good as I thought or was I just easily impressed with simple, supervised walks? The true test was here for the both of us. My driver from the school shook my hand, handed me my bag, scratched Gambit's head, waved down a skycap and drove off.

This was not the medium-sized Oklahoma City airport. This was the real deal: big, loud and busy with all the good distractions a large airport has to offer. As we followed the skycap to our gate, Gambit was awesome. He was smooth, fluid and focused as we maneuvered together through this first true, real-world test. The test was on me—the dog was performing A+. I can always tell when the guide is focused and attentive by the way he's moving at a quick pace and pulling into the harness. These dogs love to work and Gambit was clearly in his element.

We arrived at the gate, thanked the skycap, checked in and sat down. No big deal; just a couple of pros at this guide dog thing. The airline stewards allowed us to pre-board a few minutes ahead of the crowd so we could get situated. They put us in the bulkhead as it has more legroom, with space to give the dog a little more room to lie down. These dogs are trained to work themselves under the seat the best they can, curl tight and lay still. Most fellow passengers walking down the aisle don't even know the dog is onboard until we unload. I normally get plenty of compliments and positive comments. I also soon noticed the dog is a nice ice-breaker for those around me. I like this, as it makes what could be an awkward situation turn into a friendly conversation. Most people seem to like dogs and the idea of being around a guide dog is a "conversation piece" in almost all situations.

I hadn't really thought about how the public would react to a dog being present, often in close quarters on planes, buses, in restaurants, offices and other places. I'd say it's 99 percent positive and welcoming. Federal law allows for the access of service animals to be accepted into any business open to the public. For the one-percenters who act like I'm not welcome, I "educate" them and take my business elsewhere. Even though we are allowed in all public places, it is suggested by the school to not take the dogs to a zoo (the residents might get a little excited) and movie theaters (not even a dog wants to lay on those floors).

As our plane arrived in Oklahoma City, I remember the man of the hour was not me but Gambit, as it should be. He was not just a new family member and friend; his amazing talents were an integral part of how I would continue this new phase of my life.

As we made our move to Tulsa in the next few weeks, all was good. Pat had no trouble finding a new teaching position, we found good childcare for Matt, and I started my job on July 1, 1987. What had just happened? The previous 16 months had come and gone through the churning gears of losing my sight, testing my faith, stumbling with a cane, learning to stay positive, losing a job, getting a job, surviving Kansas City with Big Dave, disliking a rehab center, loving a rehab center, boxing up an old way of life and unboxing a new one.

All in all, things seemed to be working.

I'm not sure I ever took a city bus prior to losing my sight, but I knew utilizing the public transit system for my job would allow me to be less dependent on others. Most city buses are designed to route themselves to a downtown station, which made getting to my downtown Tulsa office the simple act of getting on and off one bus. With stopping and starting at traffic lights every block, going up or down certain mild elevations or dips in the streets and making multiple turns along my bus route, I was able to quickly get a feel of my location in the downtown area at any given time. It was fairly easy to know when to get off, and most drivers were pretty good at remembering where Gambit and I were supposed to exit.

Starting the job was a dual education. I needed to learn the natural gas marketing business and I also had to learn to work on a computer. The computer and I were in this together, so we had to learn to get along. This was well before the Internet, so that type of digital transfer of information and connectivity was several years in the future. I depended on my newly learned computer skills for such basic day-to-day things as a phone list, calculating transactions, drafting letters and agreements, reading and storing documents, creating cheat sheets on computer commands, the football schedule for my Sooners and typed work notes.

Robert Hutton was true to his word, and the talking screen-reader adaptation to a desktop computer was waiting on me when I arrived. The first couple of days, a computer company representative conducted training. Robert also made arrangements for Pat, Matt and me to travel to the screen-reading manufacturing company's head office in Florida for a week of personalized training. Robert went above and beyond in giving me every opportunity to be successful within the company, Hutton Gas. I felt very, very lucky to have crossed paths with him.

Technology has certainly advanced since my first talking screen-reader computer in 1987. It was a large, klutzy speaker plugged into a desktop computer that only managed to work effectively with basic word-processing and spreadsheet applications. Now there is a software application that can work with any computer, including laptops, that uses the Windows operating system; no external hardware is necessary. Today's screen-reader software costs about one-fifth of those early voice products.

"Voiceover" functions now can be installed on Apple smart phones and tablets to provide a voice telling the user what appears on the screen. With his fingertip, the user can "flick" to the left or right to maneuver throughout apps on the device. There are also websites that allow me to download audible books and magazines to my iPhone. I would assume most, if not all, textbooks are available for visually impaired students. This was not possible before the digital age of the last 10-15 years. I now read books all the time and this is another great tool to be connected to the "real" world.

You guessed it—when I started at Hutton's company, my ten thumbs made my computer training a little more of an adventure than I would have hoped, but I stuck with it despite a test of my patience. As time went on, the computer skills kicked in and I got up to speed on learning the job. With my landman background and overall basic understanding of the oil and gas industry, Robert's assumption was right: it was a natural transition for a land-man into this new work in gas marketing.

Again, it seemed I was surrounded by good people.

It turned out that one of the new employees at the company was a guy I knew from college. He wasn't in the gas-marketing group, but we ran into each other most days. His wife and Pat were sorority sisters, so not only was it nice to know someone within the company, but it also made it easier to get reacquainted with some of their current Tulsa friends whom we knew from college. This guy was pretty clever and tried to help me with various ways of getting around the office and improvising ways to learn and do my job. One day, he showed up with a map of the state of Oklahoma. He had taken a seamstress sewing wheel with a perforated edge and outlined each county by rolling the wheel along the county boundary from the backside of the map. This acted like braille tactical bumps on the face of the map, and enabled me to identify the shape and boundary of each county so I could place braille labels in the center of each county. This process made it easier to visualize the locations of various counties when discussing the building of a gathering system for gas production or talking with a client about specific areas around the state. The sewing wheel probably looked odd sitting on my desk, but it was effective and useful in many ways.

Much of my job was done on the phone—calling on clients, building rela-tionships, negotiating deals, sharing market intelligence and working out var-ious issues. This worked out really well for me. After all, one cannot recognize a blind guy from the opposite end of the phone. The subject of my blindness never came up in business conversations over the phone. Why would it? Sure, I had to conduct my work a little differently to adapt, and so did most of my co-workers around me, but what did blindness have to do with getting to know a customer, identifying his or her needs, negotiating a transaction, convincing this customer to do my deal or discussing each other's background, family or college football? Did I sound blind on the phone? Of course not.

I loved the job, enjoyed learning more about the gas marketing business and getting to know the people, co-workers and clients. Not all was great, as many frustrations would come and go, both in the job and with normal daily tasks, but I was so thankful to be on my feet and being productive.

As the months went by, I gained confidence, not only in my work but also in my ability to work around the blindness. Gambit and I were a good team and we trusted each other to get around downtown. I joined professional associations and business groups and attended monthly meetings. I could always find the location of the buildings and would normally ask an acquaintance to meet me at the street-level door of the meeting place so we could walk in together.

Gambit always seemed to be a reliable spark to conversation. Most people naturally like dogs and are genuinely interested in guide dogs. I learned that when I went inside a restaurant, a host or hostess would typically say, "Hello" or "Welcome" or "Can I help you?" This enabled me to locate the hostess stand, announce that I was meeting someone and ask, "Could you go ahead and seat me?" This way, I could get situated with Gambit lying closely next to me, making himself as small as possible. I would then be ready to offer a handshake when the client showed up. I found this to be a comfortable way to meet the client. I could introduce the dog in a conversational way, already be seated and, by the end of the lunch, everyone was comfortable. When the waiter came with the check, I made a point to hand my credit card directly to the waiter, since I didn't know for sure where the check might be set down. I would then ask the client to write a tip on the ticket, help me put my finger on the X to sign, and off we would go. It worked.

Fast-forward three months after moving to Tulsa. I walked in our house after work one evening and Pat announced, "I'm pregnant."

"Who said that? Who's out there!? I just started a new job. You just started a new job. We live in a small two-bedroom rented patio home."

Those were the things I wanted to say, but instead offered: "How exciting. How did that happen?"

I accompanied Pat to most of her obstetrician appointments. Dr. Patricia Daily was great, and one day she said, "I think when the baby's arrival day gets here, you should have Gambit in the delivery room. I'll talk to the hospital staff to make sure it's okay. How's that sound to you, Dad?"

"OK with me," I said. "That'll be a first." Actually, my initial thought was: "If it's a 20-hour labor, where will I take Gambit out to relieve?" I doubted the hospital staff had signed up for that one.

Pat was due on July 11, 1988. For some unknown reason, she thought it would be a good idea to invite some friends and family over for a July 4th party on the evening of the 3rd. A few friends lingered around the party until about 10:00 p.m., when Pat announced she was tired and needed to get to bed. I stayed up a little later, finally ushering our friends out the door about midnight.

At about 4:00 a.m., Pat lovingly nudged me—a hard elbow to my ribs—and said, "I think my water broke. We need to get to the hospital!"

The plan went into action. A neighbor came over to stay with three-year-old Matt while my mom came to transport Pat, me and Gambit to the hospital. We arrived at 4:45 and things started happening very quickly. The attendant put Pat in a wheelchair and hustled us all to a room. We got Pat in bed and Gambit in the corner, and immediately it was all-hands-on-deck, as Pat was very serious about her present condition.

I was trying to stay out of the way when I heard a nurse say, "Mom, you're doing great. Dad, you don't look so good. You'd better sit down." My four hours of sleep and the urgency of what was happening about took me down.

At 5:30 a.m., Dr. Daily came running in, tossed her purse somewhere in the corner and said, "Ted, get that gown and those rubber gloves on."

"Huh?"

"You're catching this kid when he or she comes out!"

"What kid?"

"Get over here!"

Boom. Done. Son Luke was born on July 4. I did catch him coming out and I was thankful for the doctor's idea. You don't have to see to bring a child into this world.

Everyone came through with flying colors, including Gambit, and the nurse gave Pat a new nickname: "One-push Pat." Clearly, the Hinson train was rolling down the tracks, and I felt like a mere passenger. I hoped God, and not some jokester, was the conductor.

As our first year in Tulsa concluded, all was good. I was very fortunate to have been given a door-opening job by Robert Hutton. I found it easy to appreciate all the things I had, and wasn't worried about those I didn't. My job, my family and my life were going well and I had much to be thankful for. I found it easy to stay positive and motivated to be the best I could be. I wanted to be successful but was aware I had a long way to go. But so far, so good.

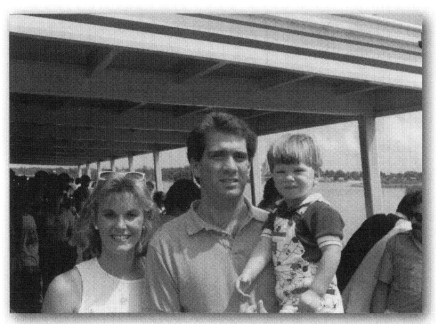

Pat, Ted and Matt, Florida, August 1987

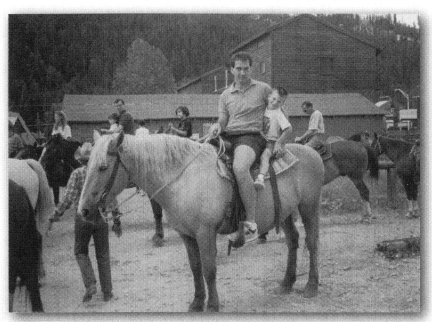

Ted and Matt, Red River, New Mexico, July 1991

9

A Bite Out of Life

Sometime during that first summer in Tulsa, a college buddy called and said, "Hey, I've got a boat and I want to take you waterskiing. How about this Saturday? Unless you're chicken!"

Kevin Ray had not changed since the good old fraternity days. This is the way he always got his friends to go have some fun.

"Great, can't wait!" I lied.

I had water-skied growing up, so I wasn't so worried about attempting this activity, but I was concerned about the stupidity/danger factor. I needed to come up with a simple plan to keep me out of harm's way on the water.

On that Saturday morning before Kevin, his wife Lee, and our friends Ed and Julie Roberts showed up to pick us up for the drive to the lake, I had made my simple plan. First, I had Pat go out and find a kid's whistle. Then I told her, "When I get up on the skis and feel confident enough to cut outside the wake, I'll point either to the right or left. If it's clear, blow the whistle once; if it's not clear, blow the whistle twice. That will be my signal to make an outside move or not. Whatever you do, do NOT let Ed have the whistle."

I remembered my basic waterskiing lessons taught by my Uncle Joe when I was 12 years old: Keep the skis up, knees tucked, lean back, hold on and let the boat do all the work. So, out of the water I came and it felt pretty cool, just like old times. I heard all the whooping and hollering from the boat. Good stuff. I remember feeling thankful for having friends to suggest these things to get me out and have some fun.

I hung on for a while and felt pretty comfortable. It wasn't long before I thought, "It's time to get out of my comfort zone and try to cut outside the wake." I instinctively knew that when I approached the wake, the surface elevation of the water would change, and this sensation alone might be enough to cause me to go down. Still, this wouldn't be the first time I embarrassed myself in front of these old friends. Other thoughts ran through my head: "Can I trust Pat's judgment with the whistle signal? Can I trust Kevin's boat-driving skills or his assessment of potential danger? Are they taking this situation as seriously as I am? Do they even really like me?"

I knew there was only one way to find out. I pointed to the right and waited for Pat to blow one or two blasts—the clear or not-clear signal. Instead, I heard three distinct whistles.

"Crap! Ed has the whistle. Screw it. Here I go." And out I went. I'm sure I looked like an old man, scared to death and hanging on for dear life. But nothing ventured, nothing gained. I avoided disaster and had a great experience.

It was a wonderful day—good times with good friends, but also, in a bigger way, a day of learning to trust those around me and being treated in a "normal" way. I realized this was the new normal for me. If I were to enjoy what life had to offer, I needed to learn not only how to do things differently, but also to trust myself and those around me. To take a bite out of life, we all need to push ourselves, learn to trust our untapped abilities, trust the judgment of those on our team, and then go for it.

My boss, Robert Hutton, who also lived in our neighborhood, approached me one day and asked if I ever ran for exercise. I told him I used to go for a two- or three-mile run when we lived in Oklahoma City, but I really hadn't worked out much since moving to Tulsa. He said he'd been running for about a year and asked if I wanted to go for a run. He showed up the next evening with a short piece of rope, about a foot long, with a loop tied on each end. We each stuck a finger in our end of the rope and away we went.

As we slowly jogged along, I noticed I had to be very conscientious about keeping my feet up, not getting lazy or tired and shuffling or dragging them. It wouldn't take much to trip over a small lip in the path or shuffle my feet over a slight rise of elevation on the pavement. If I did, I could go down in a hurry. Robert learned to tell me of large cracks or lips in the road, to avoid running up or down curbs, and to watch out for low-hanging branches. It was a lot like guide-dog work, just not as professional.

We began running several times a week and eventually got up to four or five miles per run. We soon traded in the thicker rope for a thin, leather boot-lace. I know we turned some heads, and occasionally we'd get asked about the purpose of the rope. I really didn't care for getting this attention; one of us would just reply that I was visually impaired. I did enjoy being outside and running. It was the exercise I needed to stay in shape and it served as a great stress reliever.

After we'd been running together for a few months, Robert said, "The Tulsa Run is in a couple of months and I'm thinking about doing it. Why don't you do it with me?"

Well, there were many good reasons to not do that run. First, it was 9.3 miles long, which seemed like a long way. The Tulsa Run is a big deal for Tulsans, with thousands of people training for it every year. Robert and I had our comfortable four- or five-mile route around our neighborhood or along the nearby Arkansas River trail, but the Tulsa Run was a whole different ball-game. It would be packed with runners, elbow to elbow, and with our running side-by-side with our tether, we would be a double-wide. But I overcame those reservations and concluded that it definitely would be a nice challenge and a heck of a goal.

I knew lots of friends who had done the Tulsa Run—some avid, competitive runners who do it most years, and some who just set a goal to finish it one time and check it off their list. I figured I'd run it once and then decide if it would become a tradition.

The big run day came and it was even more crowded than I had anticipated. There were runners of all shapes and sizes, with lots of pre-race laughter and fun. I recall there were almost 8,000 runners that year, which is about normal. We made the strategic error of starting near the back where it wasn't so crowded. I thought this would allow us to have a little elbow room and allow the crowd to thin out so we could maneuver our double-wide frame. Unfortunately, it never thinned out like we'd hoped because the crowd was just too big. As we worked around a few slower-paced people, others with a naturally slower pace always seemed to be ahead of us. There just weren't very many "passing lanes" for our wide load.

But the good news was that these issues caused us to relax into a slower pace and not feel like we had to overdo it, which was fine. It was obvious early on, with the rookie mistake of starting in the back, that we were not going to have a great time, speed-wise, on this adventure.

Over the years, I ran several Tulsa Runs with different running buddies. I learned I had no reason to have an ego when it came to this event. I'm an average runner and, after a couple of times, no matter what my training regimen or how much we pushed it on race day, my time was always within a few minutes of the previous race. So, my attitude was just to enjoy the event and feel good about knocking it out as a nice accomplishment.

After I'd been running about three or four years, I had another buddy suggest we do the Tulsa Triathlon.

"Okay, now you're getting a little extreme," I responded.

Pat and I owned an old-school, three-speed tandem bicycle to cruise around town. He suggested we'd train on it, and then on race day we'd rent a nice race bike. So, the run part was no big deal and we had the bike part figured out, but what about the swimming part? Well, the swimming leg would prove a little tricky. First of all, I'm a terrible swimmer, with or without vision. I don't have good form, I'm not very buoyant and I basically hate it. I trained in an indoor pool with lanes separated by roped floats. On race day, our plan was to have a partner in a row boat call out and give me a general idea where I was going while my race buddy swam at my side.

The swim part was the first leg of this adventure. We arranged with the race organizers to allow me to start my swim 15 minutes before actual race time. This would allow us to avoid the big crowd of swimmers at the start and not get in the way of the real triathletes. As we zig-zagged the one-mile course across Lake Keystone, the swimmers gained on me. When we got within a hundred yards of the swim finish, Paul the boatman yelled (lied): "You only have twenty yards to go; kick it in gear!" I did, kind of, and got out of the water only seconds before the lead swimmers. My son Matt, then five years old, thought I won the swim leg. He was so proud.

Top to bottom, this was basically a stupid idea, and poorly executed—everything from the laughing/hollering rowboat guy to riding a bike we were not familiar with (and which we did not pre-check; we had to stop and fix a busted chain within one mile of the beginning of the bike leg) to telling some friends what I was doing so they could show up to witness this fiasco.

Check triathlon off the list.

I got a call from my friend David Reeves one Monday morning, two days after I had just completed another Tulsa Run. Dave had formerly lived in Tulsa and participated in a few Tulsa Runs himself. After moving to Houston, he had kept up with his running but, like me, is a big guy who isn't what you'd call a "natural" runner.

He said, "Hey, let's do the Houston Marathon."

"Are you nuts?" I laughed. I honestly thought he was joking, maybe making fun of my recent Tulsa Run time.

"No. It's a big deal down here: Thousands of runners, bands playing, usually 100,000 fans along the way rooting runners on. Come on, it'll be cool. You can tell your grandkids one day."

"No way," I told him. "You're biting off more than you can chew on this one. Those are real runners. I've heard stories about marathon runners passing out, getting hauled off on a gurney, losing control of their bladders and other bodily functions. Why would you want to put your body through that, especially in public?"

Dave was persistent. "Hinson, let me tell you about those guys," he said. "They have those problems because the week of the marathon, they change what they eat, how they run, how they sleep—all that stuff. I'm not going to change anything—not what I eat, how I run or my brand of cigarettes!"

This was the first week of November and the Houston Marathon was in January.

"We don't have the time to train!"

"We can just fake it and see what happens race day," were his final words of encouragement.

"OK, the answer is still no, but I'll train for six weeks and see how it goes," I said.

A couple of my running buddies in Tulsa had just done a marathon a month or so before, so I asked them if they wanted to do some long runs with me. They were in good shape and decided not only to train with me but also go to Houston to run the marathon, too. We did cram the training into the next two months and, unfortunately, I didn't get injured. I had no excuse to not do this marathon.

Marathon day arrived and we were pumped up—and also scared to death. What had we gotten ourselves into? Oh sure, I can pretend to have a good attitude, preach my motivation and stay positive, but this is a marathon, for crying out loud—a 26.2-mile nightmare on feet. So much for acting like no big deal and thinking positive; this would be a mountain of physical agony— on display for thousands in Houston to witness.

We somehow survived it. I hated it and I loved it. I thought it was the dumbest and most fun thing I've ever done. I told the guys I did two marathons in one day: my first and my last.

At this point, in the mid-1990s, we had a running group of six or seven guys who met at my house three or four times per week. We weren't hardcore runners. We enjoyed just doing our regular runs, no keeping time or pushing each other along. We would stop and get water, talk, and if someone was having a slow day, one guy would always hang back with him. We'd all just take it easy. No reason for anyone to pretend to have an ego in this group. But one day, one of the guys got the itch and started to talk about a marathon, so most of us took the bait. We decided to do the Chicago Marathon in October of 1996. It was about six months away, so we'd have time to properly train and prepare for a weekend in a fun city.

About six of us made the trip and all went well. The Chicago Marathon experience was both terrible and great—again, love and hate—but the hot, hot tub afterwards hurt so good. Nothing like lots of pizza after a marathon for dinner, starting with onion rings as an appetizer and whatever cake a la mode was offered for dessert.

I'm sure that for my "pilots," doing these long runs with me is a challenge in itself—watching out for irregular surfaces, overhangs, maneuvering the both of us around all sorts of objects, some stationary and some moving, not to mention the pilot's own effort to do his run. I'm sure it can be taxing and I've always appreciated this effort.

My friend, Craig, was in town over a Thanksgiving weekend visiting family, and he called me Thursday morning.

"Hey, I saw in today's paper there's a three-mile run down at the river. Let's go do it."

I'd never run with Craig, which really didn't matter, but I was curious because he's a pretty big boy, "OK, but I didn't know you've been running."

"Yeah, I've run a little lately. Let's take the wives and kids and go down there."

I soon discovered he had not been running. About halfway through this three-mile run, he was hurting.

"Slow down, slow down," he gasped. "Let's take it easy."

Any slower and it would've been declared an old lady walk.

"It's OK, we're good," I told him, trying to be encouraging. "You're fine. It's mental, all mental. We can do this."

"This is not mental. I'm dying here."

The wives and kids were at the finish line cheering us on. As we approached the finish, I felt like I was pulling the tether like a leash on a stubborn Labrador. As soon as we crossed the finish, Craig heads off to the side, drops to all fours in the grass and it's upchuck time. Welcome back to Tulsa! When we all finished laughing, we felt sorry for the guy.

A couple of years later, the same "runner" friend phoned and suggested: "Let's take the boys snow skiing. I'm taking my son, John is taking both of his boys, so you should join us and take Matt and Luke. It'll be a blast and good experience for the kids. You'll be fine; I'll act as your guide."

"So, Craig, have you been skiing lately?" I asked, not expecting to get an honest answer.

"Sure, no problem."

"Okay, I'll check with the boys. And I think I'll check on getting a trustworthy guide from the ski area."

This was probably the biggest combination of excitement, nerves, doubt, exhilaration, trust and fear I can think of. I only skied once before losing my sight, so I knew better than to pretend like it was no big deal and feel overly confident. I knew if things got ridiculously stupid and disastrous, then I'd sit it out and let my boys enjoy the trip with their friends. The guide strongly recommended I wear a vest that read "Blind Skier" while he wore a "Blind Guide" vest. This, I'm sure, was a great idea to give everyone a heads-up and give me a little more space to tumble and fall. The guide followed me down, staying close behind—untethered—and issuing verbal commands, e.g.," Stay right. Easy to the left. Let 'em run. We're going to stop in thirty yards so listen up."

Getting on the chairlift was an adventure in itself. You get one shot, and if you don't time it right and get on that seat, it's all over, so get out of the way and try again. I went snow skiing two or three times and each time came home humbled, yet in one piece.

When I've done stuff like a marathon or the triathlon or snow skiing, some people might think, "He's just showing us a blind guy can do this, proving a point." Well, that's not it, at least not for me. That's not what motivates me to do some of these things. These are physical, fun challenges many people do all the time. "Because you can" is a typical reason to do any of these things. Sure, it's nice to set a goal, go do it, and then feel good about it, as you should. The reason I do these things is because they are a part of enjoying all parts of life, challenging yourself. I would've done them if I had my sight. Why not? It's about taking a bite out of life!

I value Mark Twain's quote: "Twenty years from now, you will be more disappointed by the things that you didn't do than by the ones you did do."

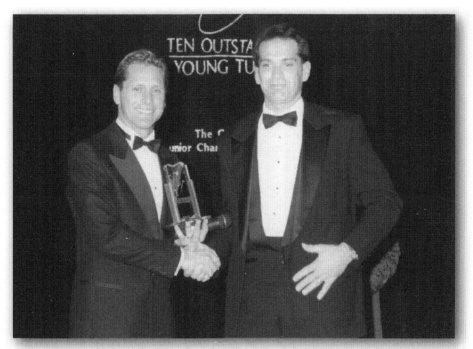

Ted receiving "Ten Outstanding Tulsans Award" with Steve Largent, 1996

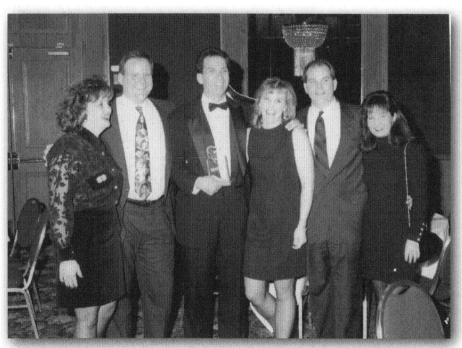

Ten Outstanding Tulsans Award Dinner with friends, Julie Roberts,
David Reeves, Ted, Pat, Craig Ferguson, Nancy Ferguson, 1996

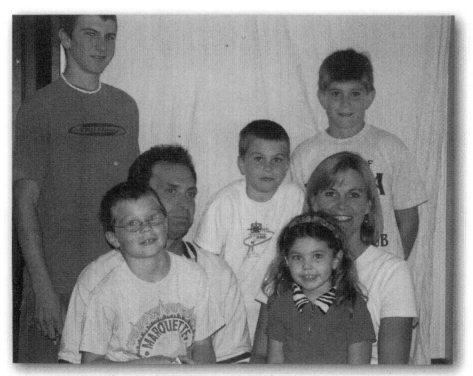

Daniel, Anna, Ted, Pat, Matt, Samuel, Luke, Summer 1999

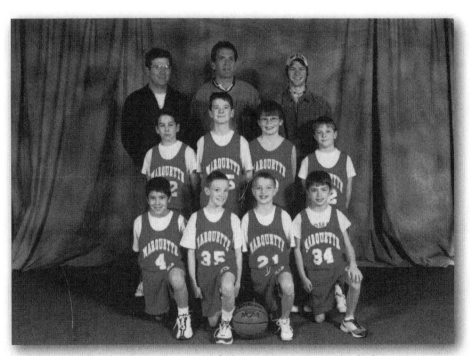

Coaches James Barnes, Ted Hinson, Matt Hinson with the
Marquette School 3rd Grade basketball team, 2002

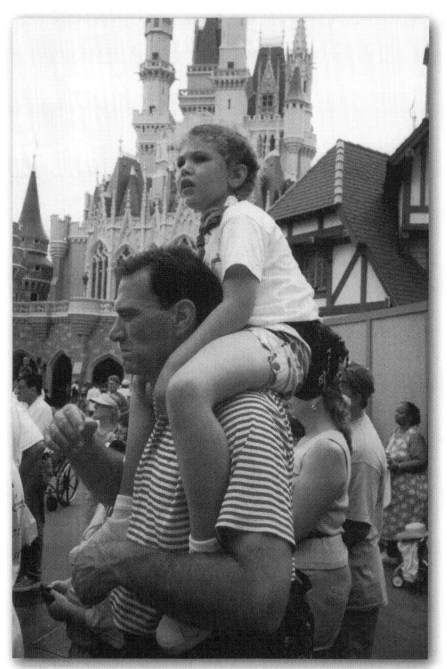

Ted and Anna, Disneyworld, 2002

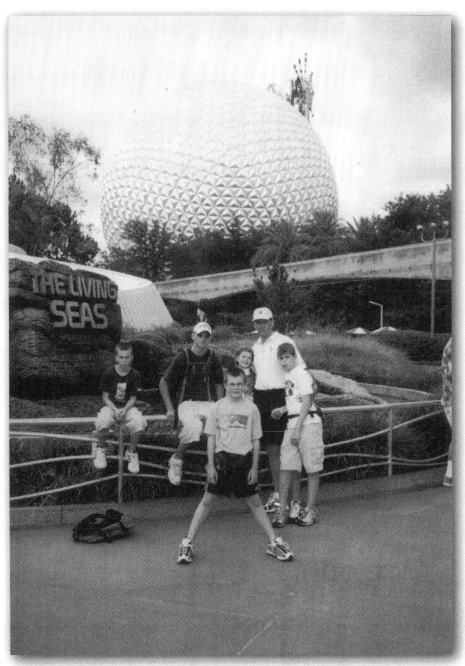

Samuel, Matt, Anna, Ted, Luke, Daniel, Disneyworld, 2002

10

My Normal

In the spring of 1990, Pat and I decided to take a trip to Medjugorje, Yugoslavia (a country now known as Bosnia and Herzegovina). Since 1981, visions of the Virgin Mary have been seen by six local teenagers in this town in the southwest part of the country. Many Christians, both Catholic and Protestant, have traveled to Medjugorje as a pilgrimage and religious retreat. We had learned about the miracles at Medjugorje only a few months prior to planning this trip, but we felt it was something we really wanted to do. Mom had welcomed the idea of keeping Matt and Luke over the ten-day trip, so we finalized arrangements with a group from Tulsa.

Many people travel all around the world for miracles. I'm sure some seek specific physical healings and others feel it necessary to visit these spiritual locations for reasons they can't explain. I am sure many prayers are answered and miraculous physical healings occur at these spiritually touched places, but these were not the reasons we chose to go to Medjugorje. Pat and I had not traveled much, especially out of the country, so the thought of an international trip was exciting in itself. But the Catholic overtone of daily Mass, Bible readings, testimonials, learning regional religious history and traveling with this good group of 20 people from Tulsa were reasons far beyond just going on a nice journey.

To be quite honest, I've never spent a lot of time praying for God to heal me of my blindness. Don't get me wrong—I've prayed for many things directly and indirectly related to my loss of vision, and I'd certainly welcome regaining my sight, either from a sudden miracle from God or through a medical breakthrough involving the rejuvenation of dead nerve tissue. Some people may think I don't have enough faith, I'm not praying enough, I've given up on prayer or become apathetic. Well, they can think that, but they would be wrong. God knows me, He knows my needs and listens to my wants. He wants the best for me and I trust Him. He's heard my prayers and He has a plan. This is what I know.

Something else I know is that I have a life to live and things to do, kids to raise, a wife to love, a career to grow, a community to become involved in and friends to be friendly with. Maybe someday, either by God blessing me directly or blessing a doctor who treats me, it might happen, but I can't sit around and fret about it. I choose not to ride that emotional roller coaster.

The trip to Yugoslavia was amazing. The Tulsa priest who accompanied our group, Fr. Robert Dubrowski, had survived the Dachau concentration camp during World War II, and this in itself was an inspirational part of our trip. Learning the Yugoslavian history, visiting the religious shrines, attending Mass in a foreign country and being present with thousands of Godly followers from around the world was incredible and impactful. We climbed up mountains for midnight prayer service, attended religious talks and just absorbed the spiritual environment.

Once I arrived in Medjugorje, for some reason my prayer during the trip seemed to be focused on contentment. I felt thankful for all I had, didn't dwell on what I had lost, but prayed for the stability of contentment—not so content that I lacked ambition or drive, but accepting of the realistic restrictions I had and continuing to try to be successful with whatever situation I'm in at that time, with the immediate priorities of both family and work, and just being the best I can be for now.

The trip was great in all aspects. We arrived back in Tulsa, back into the real world, and our spiritual tanks were full.

About two months later, the Hutton company was enduring a rough time. Some jobs were lost and other jobs were becoming shaky. Bankruptcy was being discussed. I approached Robert and told him I was absolutely loyal and appreciative of his giving me this job and I was willing to ride it out.

"Ted, I appreciate that," he said, "but this thing might not end well for anyone. Do yourself a favor and look around and do what you have to do. I promise I'll understand."

Paul Brothers, one of the guys in my Bible study, talked to a golfing buddy of his who was vice president of Vesta Energy Company, a mid-size natural gas marketing company in Tulsa. "You need to call David Tudor at Vesta," Paul advised.

I contacted him that day. "David, this is Ted Hinson. Paul suggested I give you a call about coming in and discussing a gas marketing position."

"Yes, Paul said you'd be calling me. Sounds like you've been doing gas marketing for about three years. Can you come in next week for an interview?"

"Yes, thanks. I appreciate it. Did Paul mention my vision problem?"

"What vision problem?" David said.

"Well, I've got…"

David cut me off. "Yes, he mentioned that. No problem. We'll see you next week."

I began working for Vesta in the summer of 1990. It was a good company with lots of good people about my age who liked to work hard and play hard. I quickly realized I had gained good experience and learned a lot from working at Hutton. What a relief! Vesta was a bigger company with many meetings, lots of transactions, lots of clients and contacts in their business network. I had a ton more to learn and it was exciting. All was good.

"Ted, I'm pregnant," Pat said as I walked in from work one evening, a few months after joining Vesta.

I guess this was the normal course of life for people our age: buy a house, have a kid, sell a house, buy a house, have another kid, start a new job, clip coupons for diapers, make more friends, get involved in the church—all that good stuff. Other than getting a new guide dog occasionally, I guess this was just everyday life.

Samuel was born in September 1991. All went well, but Gambit did not make the delivery this time; his one experience was plenty for all. As with Luke, I got to catch Samuel coming out and the delivery was a piece of cake (easy for me to say). Samuel started sleeping through the night within the first week of coming home from the hospital. Thank you, God.

One afternoon, Pat was taking a nap with Samuel, so I thought I'd take three-year-old Luke for a walk around the block. We had a backpack built for carrying a toddler. It had a metal frame and could hold about 50 pounds. I walked out to the garage with Luke in hand, let him go and pushed the garage door opener. As I grabbed the backpack off the hook on the garage wall, I heard, "Daddy, Daddy. Help, Daddy!" What the heck? I hustled across the garage to the sound of Luke's desperate yell. As I got closer, I could tell his yelling was coming from about my head level, maybe six feet off the ground. Luke had grabbed the bottom handle of the garage door as it was raising up, overcommitted and was hanging onto the handle with both hands in a death grip. I should've left him there!

I got him down, stuffed him into the backpack and off we went. I made a mental note to watch out for that situation again. It could've been ugly.

Samuel was only seven months old when Pat made a familiar announcement: "Hi, Honey. How was work? I'm pregnant."

"Well, of course you are."

At this point, bring it on. All three boys were healthy and, apparently, we were meant to have a big family. Daniel was born in February 1993. He didn't start sleeping through the night as quickly as Samuel did, unfortunately. After ten months of his waking up and screaming each night, he finally slept through the night. Thanks a lot, God.

The job was going well. The staff at Vesta was always supportive and worked with me when necessary to go over written documents such as contracts and proposals. I was thankful for the job and appreciative of the daily assistance along the way, so it was easy for me to have a positive attitude and enjoy my work. I had several co-workers comment about how my attitude was rubbing off on others around the office. I think people just like to be around positive, grateful people who like what they're doing, where they're doing it and whom they're doing it with.

I never really need the use of the guide dog around the office. I learn the layout, the location of everyone's office and where the restroom and coffee pot are, so co-workers often comment that they sometimes forget I'm blind, which I guess is a compliment. Their treating me normal is evident when someone leaves a file drawer out. Ouch!

At Vesta, it was important to get out and meet the clients and business associates. I'd take three or four business trips per year, sometimes with co-workers and other times solo, with just me and the dog. Most of our trips were to Houston, as it was the hub of the energy industry, home to most of our clients and offered other business opportunities. When I flew solo, the flight attendants and skycaps were normally very helpful. Getting off the plane was no big deal—just go with the flow, listen for a busy gate desk, ask for the assistance of a skycap, then go out to the taxi stand. I had a favorite hotel in Houston that had three main benefits: it was nice enough to invite business people over for breakfast, lunch or dinner; there was a grassy area for the dog to discreetly relieve himself; and I could manage to come and go independently. These things were important to me because it made travel less of an ordeal. Plus, the hotel doormen were always very helpful. Trust me, when a tip is involved, they can be very accommodating.

I got to know both clients and competitors pretty well. We attended many trade shows around the country. I took the guide dog on most trips, but not all. During a trade show or an outing, I did my best to not have the dog become the center of attention, but many times he did. This was fine because he was a nice icebreaker and maybe more interesting than my small talk. I know that being around the dog can be a little awkward for some people, so I always appreciated being invited to boondoggles put on by other companies. Sometimes the dog would go and sometimes not, but it always seemed that most people were kindly accommodating.

I was invited by another marketing company for a whitewater rafting trip in the Royal Gorge in Colorado. Gambit didn't make this trip: a three-day adventure with twelve people sleeping in nice, four-star tents at a campsite somewhere along the Arkansas River. We had two rubber boats with a guide in each. The sensation was unique due to the constant, second-by-second, dramatic changes in the water—smooth, slow, very fast, rough, a plunge, rough, then smooth again. I obviously wasn't there for the scenery, but it was a really cool experience with all the sudden changes and letting Nature move our boat down the river. I acted cool but I was secretly hoping that our guide was good at what he was doing, as these waters were very powerful. I may have benefited from not knowing exactly what was ahead, which is why I stayed prepared, on guard, and sat up strong in place. When the water appeared smooth for a long distance, I think the other passengers let their guard down because, in a matter of seconds, the water would turn crazy and bodies started falling all over the place. I remember thinking: "What am I going to do if everybody gets thrown out of this boat?"

And, yes, I'd go on golfing outings, because that's what you do in the oil business. I'd hit a few balls (I could tell guys just wanted to see how the blind guy can hit), but I was at my best as a passenger in the golf cart, cold drink and cigar in hand. I was actually used quite a bit to line up a putt. These golf outings were usually a "scramble" format, when all four players use the best ball hit from the spot of the last ball, so they'd have me putt first to get a line on the break of the green. Good idea, job done, now where did I put that cigar?

I got a call from a client out of Houston one day. "Hey, Ted, our company owns a hunting lodge down here in east Texas. This place is nice, not really roughing it. We've got a deer hunt planned next month, so come join us."

"Like with a gun, my finger on the trigger?"

"Well, yeah, we'll be hunting with rifles, but you can just come down and hang out around the guys and enjoy the trip. You'll like this place. Lots of good food."

Okay, so we get there and the host got to thinking. He had one of the ranch hands go out and find a red laser to tape to the rifle. "He'll be able to see your red dot and verbally guide you to point your rifle until the dot is on your target," he explained.

"You've got to be kidding me," I said.

"Just keep your finger off the trigger until I say so," said the ranch hand, with a chorus of agreement from my fellow "hunters."

Early the next morning, off we went. For some reason, they wouldn't let me carry my own weapon. I moved into the deer stand with the ranch hand, ever so quietly, as that's what we hunters do. After only a short while, he whispers, "Okay, we got one. Be still and quietly lift your rifle in place." Like all hunters, I put the rifle to my shoulder and, of course, put my eye to the scope to aim for my target. As my guide located my red laser dot, he said, "A little up and to the right. More right, slowly. Down a little. Back to the left. Now hold it there until I say shoot. SHOOT!"

I pulled the trigger and BANG! The next thing I heard was the gobble of an innocent, dying turkey. "Jeez, who's that? I'm sorry," I said, confused. "What happened? Is the deer gone?"

Laughing, my accomplice said, "Sorry, Ted, we're also hunting for turkeys. I got a little excited in the moment and just didn't think to tell you."

"Does this story have to make it back to the camp?"

"Absolutely!"

Well, the dot of my red laser beam did find a deer later that morning and I have the skin and antlers at home to prove it.

In the mid-90s, Vesta sold out to a company based in Houston. Our people and jobs slowly began transferring to the Houston office. I really didn't want to go there. We had family and so many good friends in Tulsa. We were active in our church and school and, overall, we were just part of a great community. Instead of having to make a decision, I was fortunate to land a natural gas marketing and trading position at Williams Companies, one of the premier corporations in Tulsa. It was an energetic and dynamic place to work—big trade floor, lots of phones, shouting of trades, buy this, sell that. Somehow the dog tucked himself sleepily under the desk each day and ignored all the craziness.

While I was working at Williams, apparently the good Lord decided that four kids just wasn't enough for us—we needed a full basketball team.

"Okay, Pat, after this one, I think corrective measures need to be taken."

"Knock yourself out," she retorted.

Anna was born in June 1995, and I kept my string going: four-for-four on catching these precious babes post-delivery. All was good.

We have had a blast raising these five beautiful kids—always busy, always crazy, and never a dull moment. We enjoyed living in a great neighborhood. Three other families on our block had a total of eight kids around our kids' ages. I distinctly remember walking home from the bus stop one evening, hearing a bunch of kids on our block yelling and playing. I was about a block away and thought, "What a great block we live on. All the neighborhood kids outside playing." As I approached our block, I realized our five kids were the only ones outside playing, making this entire racket. At that point, it dawned on me how large our family had become. Noise doesn't lie.

When the kids were young, Pat was always good at reading bedtime stories. It was wonderful, quality time and settled the kids down from another typical, hectic day. I wanted to be a part of this, so I started taking turns with Pat telling them bedtime stories. I would have two characters with rhyming names such as Rob and Bob, Tina and Nina, Jill and Bill, Jenny and Benny. When starting the story, I'd never disclose what type these two characters actually were. Sometimes they were just two kids, maybe siblings; other times they were birds, snakes, mules, etc. These stories were absolutely made up as I went along. Maybe the characters would climb onto the house, then cross the power lines, go down the sewer or fall into a mail truck, wake up in Chicago and then be homesick, then venture home. The kids would listen but keep asking, "What were they, what were they?" About five minutes into the story, I'd act like I forgot to tell them what the characters were and then finally tell them, keep rolling for a few more minutes and then wrap up the story. These stories lasted about ten minutes and the kids seemed to really enjoy the mystery and adventures. Or maybe they were just stalling before turning out the lights.

When Luke was in third grade, I volunteered to coach his basketball team. I did the same when Daniel was a third-grader. I coached each of these teams through fifth grade. I knew and loved the game of basketball and thought I could be an effective coach. I figured coaching is largely communicating, and this I could do. I had another dad assist me and we did pretty well. Sure, I couldn't see to correct sloppy mistakes or bad shooting form, but at that age, I felt it was more important to teach the game, work on fundamentals, and get each kid to recognize his strengths and weaknesses. Again, most of this was verbal, so that made me think of words would work best when trying to make a point with these kids.

I was competitive to a certain degree, as were most of these boys, and I wanted to find ways of getting each to do the best they were capable of doing.

I stressed the importance of some basics of the game, both as individuals and as a team, and then we'd just let things fall into place. Some of these basics were the importance of making strong and accurate passes, learning to dribble while looking up to see the floor, setting strong picks, being disciplined and staying in position in a zone defense, blocking out to get rebounds, forcing a ball handler to his left (which is usually his weakest dribbling side) and sticking with the three or four plays we had learned. There were always a couple of the "big" boys who wanted to keep the ball and dribble (or try to) all the way down the court. "No," I'd tell them, "get the ball to a guard and hustle down the court." I'd have my assistant give me a short play-by-play so I'd have a feel of who was getting it and who wasn't.

Actually, both teams did well all three years I coached. Of course, good talent makes any coach look pretty good. I'd do my share of "coaching" from the bench during games: "Hands up on defense. Move your feet. Block out. Strong passes. Make yourself big." You don't have to be sighted to remind your players of these fundamentals. All coaches yell these things because these basics are important and they are always applicable.

I never knew for sure, but I doubt other coaches or the referees knew I was blind. It really didn't matter. I never mentioned it, and why would I? Did it matter? Nope. We'd take the court like everybody else and play the game. We had lots of fun and lots of laughs while winning and losing together.

Whether it was raising kids, working, playing, committee work at church or just sitting in the stands watching my kids play ball, through all of life's daily duties the challenge of being blind was always present. I felt I was dealing with it the best I could, in my own way, and tried to never think of it as an excuse to not experience and enjoy a normal life. I felt I was, by nature, a positive, motivated person and pushed myself to be the best I could be. I learned early on that I could choose to be positive or choose to be negative about many things, and so many things were simply out of my control, so why choose to be negative?

Losing my sight was a tragedy, yes, but through all these years of dealing with it, nothing will ever compare to the tragedy our family experienced in September 2007.

11

A Bigger Loss

On Sunday evening, September 16, 2007, at 10:15, we had a knock at our door. I was getting ready for bed, so I threw on a T-shirt and shorts and went downstairs to answer the door, wondering who would be coming over at this time of night. Pat was at the St. John Hospital chapel for her weekly one-hour adoration of the Blessed Sacrament, which lasted from 10:00 to 11:00. Luke, now 19, was in the family room watching TV. I opened the door and it was Matt's girlfriend, Maggie, and her mother. Matt was 22 at the time.

They came in and sat down. Something was obviously very wrong. "I'm sorry, Mr. Hinson, there has been an accident," Maggie said. "I've been out of town. When I got off the plane an hour ago and turned my phone back on, I had several messages from the guys with Matt today. Matt and the guys went sailing on Grand Lake today. It was such a perfect day. They were sailing back to get off the water and the sunset was so beautiful that they decided to make one more swing around the area." While Maggie was telling this story, the shaking and tears started to build up. She was trying so hard to keep things together. "They had been drinking. Matt went to the back of the boat to go to the bathroom and the guys heard a splash. Matt fell in the water and they haven't been able to find him yet. It was dark at that point and the guys couldn't see or hear anything. They yelled and randomly threw out lifejackets. The light on the boat wouldn't work, so they used their flashlights on their phones, but no luck. They got back to shore and called the GRDA (Grand River Dam Authority) Lake Patrol and the patrol is out there still looking."

We just sat there, stunned. Pat would be home in a few minutes and I hated that she was going to walk into this situation. Luke hugged me, tears flowing, and said, "We need to call Father O'Brien."

Fr. Brian O'Brien was a young associate priest at our church, Christ The King. Fr. O'Brien had become very close to our family. He knew our kids through the many activities at our church and at Bishop Kelley High School, where our kids attended, and from several youth group mission trips around the country. He was very good with people of all ages, but Fr. O'Brien connected especially well with the high school youth. He was a great communicator, a great speaker from the pulpit who always delivered an outstanding message, and had established a real connection with the students.

When Luke said we needed to call Fr. O'Brien, my head was still spinning, trying to process this nightmare. Calling Fr. O'Brien was exactly the right thing to do at that moment and I'm thankful Luke had the presence of mind to think of him at this terrible time. Luke telephoned and Fr. O'Brien was at our house within about 15 minutes.

After Luke, Pat and I spoke to Fr. O'Brien for a few minutes, Maggie and her mom left. We felt the need to wake up the other three kids: Samuel (16), Daniel (14) and Anna (12). At this point, it was about 11:30 or 11:45 p.m. Maggie had given me the GRDA patrol officer's name and phone number. I called him and got a report: nothing yet, but they planned on searching through the night and we'd touch base in the morning.

Our family sat with Fr. O'Brien in the living room, dazed, scared and teary-eyed, not knowing if Matt had been picked up by another boat, made it to shore and passed out or what. We prayed, cried, conversed and tried to be optimistic as we sat listening to Fr. O'Brien. He was very calming and offered us much comfort. I know he was hurting inside, but instinctively knew he had to hold things together. He had known Matt very well for eight or ten years. He had worked in Matt's middle school youth group, accompanied him on high school youth group and mission trips, and even helped coach Matt's junior varsity basketball team at Bishop Kelley. They had a good relationship. It seemed that in his role as comforter he would not allow himself to break down and turn into one who needed to be comforted.

Fr. O'Brien said a few more prayers and left after an hour or two. Pat convinced the kids to go to bed. I laid on the couch, cell phone in hand, waiting on good news from the Lake Patrol. In my head, my hope was that Matt could have somehow made it to shore that night. They had been drinking, so possibly he made it to shore, crawled away from the water and passed out, maybe in tall grass or behind some trees, which is why he'd be hard to find. I figured this could be the case until maybe noon the next day. After that, the probability of receiving good news would be slight.

Pat and I waited until the next morning, Monday, at 7:00, to make a couple of phone calls. I called my sister and her husband, Toni and Tim Marlow, told them what I knew and asked them to come over soon so we could all go over and inform my mother. My mom, known as Nana, and Matt were very close and I knew this would be a heart-wrenching thing to do. I phoned a good friend I worked with and asked him to tell the office what was going on, and Pat called her school's principal and told him the same. She also called a couple of her friends. We didn't contact anyone else. This is not a call we wanted to make and it's not the type of thing anyone wants to hear.

Toni and Tim arrived at our house in less than an hour. After talking, hugging and crying, we decided to get it over with and go tell Nana. I wasn't sure how or when the news media gets their info, but assumed they would be aggressive and get information out sooner rather than later. I did not want Mom to hear anything from anyone else but us.

Pat stayed at the house to be with our kids and we headed out. Telling Mom what we knew, trying to stay hopeful, was as difficult as I had feared. Grandparents should never have to hear this type of news about a grandchild; it's just not the natural course. As grandparents, they grieve not only for themselves but also for their kids, the parents of this grandchild. I can't think of anything more difficult for an elderly person to encounter.

I suggested that Mom come back to our house with us. We arrived back home about the time a few friends were starting to show up. I phoned the Lake Patrol officer for an update. He informed me the search attempt had now turned from a "search and rescue" to a "search and recovery" mission. This was hard to hear, but there was no reason to be in denial or not deal with the reality. Again, I had in my head Matt could be passed out on the lake bank somewhere for a time, but by noon this first day, it would be time to digest the reality that the loss of our son was real.

By early that afternoon, the house was full of relatives and friends from all over. Two or three of Pat's women friends from church began organizing and coordinating everything that would help us. There was nothing they didn't think of and everything was handled amazingly. It was unbelievable. It seemed there was always one lady acting as head coordinator, clipboard in hand, taking notes, making lists of things to do and deal with. There was no way any such project could be handled in a better or more thoughtful way. The phone was ringing constantly and I noticed it was always answered on one ring by someone. Food was organized and scheduled, ice chests were prepared and filled, the house was picked up and cleaned, and paper plates, cups and utensils were acquired and arranged. The head coordinator, Katie Maguire, used her best judgment to monitor when the house was becoming too full and suggested to those people arriving that a wait outside was necessary.

That morning, our good friends Stuart and Kate Beal from Midland, Texas, called to let us know they heard the news and to offer their prayers. This conversation didn't take long before Stu and I were quite choked up. We had worked together for several years before Stu moved back home to Midland. Our families had done a lot together and he knew our kids well. Later that afternoon, I was on the back deck talking to someone when Pat came out and told me Stu and Kate had just walked in the house. Kate said when Stu got off the phone with me that morning, he told her, "We've got to go to Tulsa." They had access to a corporate jet and were at our house within a few hours. This effort showed me the heart, love and pain of such good friends. This was just an example of so much of the outpouring of love and thoughtfulness our family experienced that difficult week.

By mid-afternoon that first day, we were told there would be a prayer service that night at Christ The King. We still did not have any news about finding Matt, so hope still existed. We thought a prayer service with a few friends in a church setting was a good idea. For the most part, I wasn't real big on constantly being around a lot of people at that point, but this was how a strong, loving community supports families in need, so praying with a few friends and Fr. O'Brien seemed to be just what we needed.

That same afternoon, Pat got a phone call from her first cousin, Janet Puckett, of Edmond, Oklahoma. Janet said she had had an odd dream overnight about Pat's and Janet's parents, who were deceased. The dream didn't make any sense, and she really didn't think much about it until she received a phone call from her sister informing her about Matt being missing. The dream immediately came back to her. "I dreamed our parents were all together somewhere, just sitting around, waiting on something," Janet told Pat. "Then Dad said, 'Okay, let's go get him,' and all four of them stood up and walked away together."

Janet's dream revealed that our son Matt was met in Heaven by his Grandma and Grandpa Berry that night. I have no doubt.

When our family walked up to the front door of the church that Monday evening for the prayer service, we were met at the front door by our church youth director, Ron Tremblay. I'm sure Ron played a big part in organizing the service. Ron put his hand on my shoulder and said, "The church is completely full. It's standing-room only." This was overwhelming. How could something like this come together within one day? So strong, so powerful and so moving were the love and compassion felt by our family and, for that matter, everyone present in that church. It was so spiritual it's hard to put it into words.

I can't really say I remember the entire service. Again, this was not a funeral. Matt was still missing, so this was just a get-together to pray with us and be with our family. I was still in a daze and couldn't really focus on all that was happening. I did pick up on one thing that Fr. O'Brien said during the service, and it was all that needed to be said and prayed for: "Wherever Matt is, God is with him."

When we got home from the prayer service that night, at the end of this first day, the reality had set in and the nightmare was indeed real. Things in life can be cruel, unexplainable and painful beyond imagination. To me, the tragedy of losing my sight so many years ago was nothing compared to the tragedy I was now confronting. My wife and children were hurting, I was hurting, my mother was hurting, my siblings and their husbands and children were hurting, and this community, bigger and tighter than I ever realized, was hurting. My blindness had nothing to do with what I was going through. Most things I dealt with throughout each day over the past 21 years were managed around my lack of sight, but this "loss" had nothing to do with being blind or sighted. Anyone dealing with the magnitude of this type of tragedy was dealing with an hour-by-hour challenge of just trying to move forward, wondering if the pain will ever get better.

By the next day, Tuesday, my oldest sister and her husband, Aquina and Grant Buehrig, had flown in from Virginia. More hugs, more tears. By noon, our house was completely full of friends and family. The story had made the TV news and the media were calling. The house was full of people from morning until evening. I'm not sure how many people were in our house at any one time. Fifty? Sixty? Eighty? I have no idea; I just know our community network of church friends, college and high school friends, fraternity brothers and sorority sisters, business colleagues, Marquette School teachers, our kids' friends, old friends from Henryetta and all people in and out of our current lives were coming by to offer support and just be there during our time of need. Again, Katie, the head coordinator, managed things like she had done this many times before. I certainly hoped that this was not the case.

One day that week, Jim Langdon, Pat's cousin, came by for another visit. He told me of a book he had read by Dr. Elisabeth Kübler-Ross, a noted psychiatrist who had studied human near-death experiences. In her research, she had interviewed dozens of people of all ages who had experienced a near-death episode. Each person described traveling in a dark valley or tunnel toward a warm, radiant beam of light. In every recollection, each person described a similar experience and, in response, none wanted to come back to their earthly existence. The message: the pathway to a heavenly afterlife was just that awesome and incomparable. Matt was in a better place. The thought was very comforting to me. Things like this help us to deal with the pain of a loss and a broken heart.

About 7:30 on Thursday morning, September 20, my cell phone rang. It was the director of the GRDA, Kevin Easley. They had found Matt's body. I was glad and thankful this part of our living nightmare was finally over. We could now move towards closure and onward toward the different family we now were. Our family would never be the same. How could it? We were no longer complete; a part had been broken off and it was permanent. We would find a way to cope, but as parents and siblings, our family dynamic would be reshaped, reconfigured and patched together in a different form. The storm clouds would come and go and the pain would get better and healing would eventually take place, but life as we knew it would not be the same.

The house continued to be full and active every day that week. The funeral was scheduled for that upcoming Monday, September 24.

On Sunday, the 23rd, it was suggested we have a Mass in our home for just our extended family, about twenty of us. The furniture was rearranged in front of Fr. O'Brien's makeshift altar. It was all very intimate and very perfect. He asked if anyone wanted to say a special prayer or just had something to share. My niece's husband, trying to keep it together, said, "This family is so perfect. I just want to raise a family like this." They had only been married a few months.

Silently I recalled the "Footprints" poem, hoping and praying it was true.

The funeral that Monday morning was unbelievable. The church was packed. Space in our parish reception hall, including an audio and video feed of the funeral Mass, was arranged for the overflow. There were also loudspeakers outside the church for attendees who couldn't fit in the church or the parish hall. Marquette School was closed for the day as it was assumed all or most teachers would attend. The love and support was quite overwhelming for our family. Pat and I knew we had a lot of friends—our full house that week was evidence of this—but the number of attendees at Matt's funeral Mass was just so unbelievable to our family.

I can't say I clearly recall the entire funeral Mass. No parent should ever have to attend their child's funeral. It's just not the normal course of life. It happens, and it happens every day somewhere, and those parents, as members of that unfortunate club, experience the same nightmare. Many of the priests who had served at Christ The King over the years were present. Beautiful words were spoken in both the homily and the eulogy, perfect hymns were sung and the many, many family and friends in attendance made this a very special ceremony. I hated hearing the pain of the crying within the walls of our beautiful church. It seemed I could even hear the tears falling as friends and family were kneeling in prayer with us—hurting, grieving and, I felt, praying they could remove some of our family's pain and carry it themselves. The pain and love we all experienced was inescapable. I remember telling son Samuel to hold his Nana's arm and keep an eye on her. We walked out of the church to bury our son and try to step closer to some sort of closure and healing.

For many days or weeks or maybe a couple of years, I heard too many songs, had too many thoughts, too many memories or heard too many similar stories on TV or in books that would cause my eyes to moisten. Was this normal? I didn't know. I knew life would go on, time would pass and, with that, a healing would take place. The thoughts and tears would come and go, but time did help. Janet's dream of the grandparents going together to meet Matt on his arrival to join them in Heaven, and Jim's story of those not wanting to leave Heaven to come back to their earthly existence, continued to give me comfort that Matt was truly in a better place.

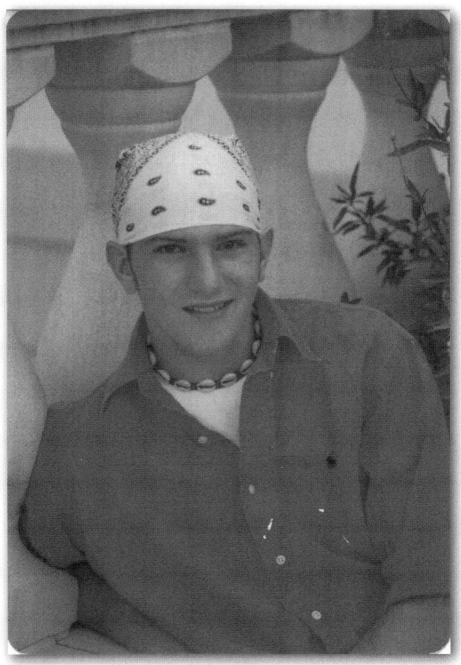

Matt, 2004

12

The Family Way

As you read through this book, you may get a feel for the day in the life of the blind, but one thing easy to overlook is the effect of those around the blind person, especially the true effect on that person's immediate family.

At the time of this writing, Pat and I have been married 34 years. Luke is 28, Samuel 25, Daniel 23, daughter Anna 21, and our deceased son Matt would have been 32. Pat prides herself on being a strong, well-rounded woman. I once heard her principal refer to her as a "locomotive"—a compliment to her strength and her teaching and administration skills at Marquette Catholic School. Please don't picture a hard, cold, steely train engine heading towards you. Pat is a determined, hard-charging, load-carrying, smiling cheerleader whom you would undoubtedly pick on your team. Luke is a rock-'em, sock-'em, loud go-getter. He loves business, the art of the deal, and his brain is always full speed ahead. Samuel is a smooth, easygoing, non-judgmental personality who likes everyone. He's a schmoozer who seemingly always has a pretty girl on his arm. Daniel is a high achiever who earned a petroleum engineering degree. In high school, he was a first team all-conference basketball player at Bishop Kelley. He aims high and stays focused. Anna, being the youngest and only girl, is the princess and, yes, after putting up with all her brothers' nonsense, she clearly deserves any special treatment she may have received along the way. She's kind and softhearted and would be the pride of any father.

Pat and I, understandably, are extremely proud of all of our kids. The three boys have all graduated from the great University of Oklahoma and Anna is in her junior year at our beloved university. These are great kids.

What was the effect of having a blind husband or father? Did things seem "normal?" I'd say that depends on your definition of "normal." Their normal is walking through a restaurant or on the beach or into a graduation ceremony with my hand on their shoulder or elbow, or sitting next to me and giving me a play-by-play of a sibling's ball game. Was this embarrassing or awkward to these kids? Maybe a little, but this was our lives and, in all honesty, aren't most teenagers embarrassed just to be in the same room with their parents, despite the circumstances? This was our normal. Sure, everyone in our family had to do some things differently at times to compensate for our different situation. This was 24/7 and the reminders were plenty.

Before the kids were of driving age, Pat had to run every errand, make every trip to the store and, when we had conflicts in our family schedule, drop me off with whatever kid at one event and speed off to another. That was our life, as parents and children, and this is how we did it all.

Being blind is a real pain in the you-know-what for me and my family unit. This is my life. This is the life of our family. We are a team, we make it work—no excuses. This is how our family gears turn. We dealt with our "normal" lives in a way I'd feel confident saying we would not change if "do-overs" were an option.

When I mention a "do-over," I mean that, in the context of my blindness being an irreversible part of our lives, we would do everything the same: the busy schedule with ballgames, school events, social activities, family vacations, etc. Sure, things on our schedule are more challenging for us with my being blind, and a simpler and easier lifestyle would be less demanding. But this is who and what we are, and the complication of blindness was not going to prevent us from visiting the places we wanted to go, doing the things we wanted to do, including the way we wanted to raise our kids. We wanted a full life and our kids wanted, and deserved, a lifestyle that fit our family persona.

I've read about and heard some people with various handicaps and hardships state that if they had a choice, they would choose to not change a thing—past, present or future. I admire this thought and attitude. I think it's remarkable, courageous and shows strong character. I've learned many, many lessons throughout blindness. It's been my life for 30 years, like it or not, but in all honesty I have to say, yes, I would certainly reverse this handicap if I could. This disability is not my choice, but we do not have the option of making a choice like this, nor can we control the exact course on our path of life.

Have these limitations restricted many things or kept things out of reach? Of course; there is no reason to deny this fact. Have these limits caused me to look deeper for other ways to live my life or create methods in order to achieve things? Absolutely. When challenged, I have improvised alternative ways to get things done, which pushed me to find strengths or capabilities that may have gone untested or remained idle. We've all heard the saying "When one door shuts, another will open." Well, when you find that alternative door, why lightly knock when a strong kick or crowbar will get the job done better? Sometimes you just need to get your attitude right and muscle things around a little.

So, what is the effect of being married to or the child of a person with this life of blindness? My wife is a special education teacher. It is her nature to support (push) those around her to be their best. Will my kids dedicate their lives to solving the needs of the disabled or possibly find a cure to blindness? Probably not. But will they subconsciously or empathetically assist those around them who need a little help? I truly believe they will. As much as anyone, they understand the real world has unique, often unforeseen challenges, and one should not use setbacks as an excuse to avoid living a fruitful, productive life.

As parents, we are teaching our children by our actions, conversations, attitudes and overall treatment of others. Our children, no matter their age, are always watching and subconsciously learning from us. This is simply human nature. If you don't think this matters, then I think you're fooling yourself. They watch and listen to all we do and say, assessing what we've done and what we've failed to do.

I mentioned earlier in this book that one of my motivating factors was always wanting to make my kids proud. This doesn't mean I'm proud of everything I've done, but I do feel I've handled my setbacks well and am living a full and fruitful life. Have I taught them well? Time will tell.

13

Not The Final Chapter

Therefore, since we have been justified through faith, we have peace with God through our Lord Jesus Christ, through whom we have gained access by faith into this grace in which we now stand. And we boast in the hope of the glory of God. Not only so, but we also glory in our sufferings, because we know that suffering produces perseverance; perseverance, character; and character, hope. And hope does not put us to shame, because God's love has been poured out into our hearts through the Holy Spirit, who has been given to us.

-ROMANS 5: 1-5

The above scripture passage really hit home for me a few years after losing my sight. It got my attention as I found myself stubbornly fighting through my blindness, taking on the challenges, being proud of the smallest of accomplishments, proving to myself that, even though I was different and had to do things differently, I held on to the confidence and belief that I would maintain as normal a life as possible. My life was what it was and I would take a bite out of it, no matter what. I would take the good with the bad, recognize the humor in certain incidents, not take myself too seriously and try to push for success and productivity in the task at hand.

As mentioned, I found motivation in two things: making my kids proud and moving forward in a positive way. Nobody said life is easy, but it's been made easier by the incredible support I've had throughout my journey of this thing called blindness, whether it is good family, supportive and caring friends, the understanding of co-workers or timely job opportunities. I have been very fortunate. When I say this, some people may reply, "Well, good people create and deserve good opportunities." This is true, in the sense that good people who work hard will have opportunities come their way. But it never hurts to be a little lucky, too. In all honesty, I consider myself lucky, and I thank God every day.

Is the above scripture true within me? Have I persevered? Do I have a strong character? I would say that I've been blessed by God and I am persevering and trying to be of strong character but, like most things, I'm a work in progress. It seems obvious to me, by fighting and managing the challenges of life, either small or large, a person will build a trait of perseverance, which will strengthen and form his or her character. I, along with my wife, have experienced a couple of rare and abnormal tragedies: a physical affliction that created the hardship of a disability and the loss of a son, which took me to the brink of emotional devastation. But I always remind myself that many people have suffered more.

Dealing with the challenges of life must be managed in the best way a person can absorb, rationalize and process. But, as I've indicated throughout this writing, I have been fortunate to be surrounded by, and connected with, many good people along the way. From the thoughtful gift of a braille watch to the getaway trip with my wife given by her sorority alumnae; from the guys' trip with Big Dave and old friends to the push by Craig and Nancy to trick me into a normal night out dancing with my wife; from the insistence of the inner-voice of an employer to say, "Yeah, let's give this guy a chance" to the blessings of five healthy kids; from the community support and strength to lift my family after losing a son to the simple, normal treatment so many people have given me over the years, I've been exceedingly blessed.

Several people have said I need to write a book: "You've got a good story—get it out there." Well, my story is somewhat unique and, I'd like to think, interesting and encouraging. But it made me think—we all have a story. Each day, week and year are additional chapters. Our story is why we are who we are, where we are and what people think of us. Our story represents our decisions, our accomplishments and shortcomings, our experiences and reactions to those experiences, the history of how we've treated people and why. We subconsciously write our story every day, for good or bad, but it represents our true lives, just not on written pages. Some of our chapters we may not be proud of or care to repeat. Our actions speak loudly and history is just that: history.

Yes, we all have a story, but it's unfinished, still an open book. Maybe we can't change the story of our past history, but anyone can control most of their remaining personal story by making good decisions, staying faithful, controlling our mouth, treating people like we want to be treated, conducting our personal and business lives in a truthful and honest way and, overall, being the best we can be. It takes work, but doesn't everything of value take hard work? A setback is just that: a setback. No reason to dwell on it or be defeated by it. It's only another chapter of who you are, not the final outcome or the end of your story.

What's your story? Are you proud of your story? If not, remember that you are in control of your actions, your remaining days and your upcoming history defined by those days. What are you going to do with it?

People along the way have said my story is inspirational or motivational. So, is this an inspirational or motivational book, like so many others? Well, if it inspires or motivates you, then that's what it is to you. But that's for each reader to judge. I hope it is helpful in a revealing sort of way. Is it humorous, sad, scary, judgmental, a testimony? Well, I might suggest it's a smorgasbord of parts of all those topics, which is what I've experienced these 30 years since I lost my sight—an exciting, interesting, almost normal life.

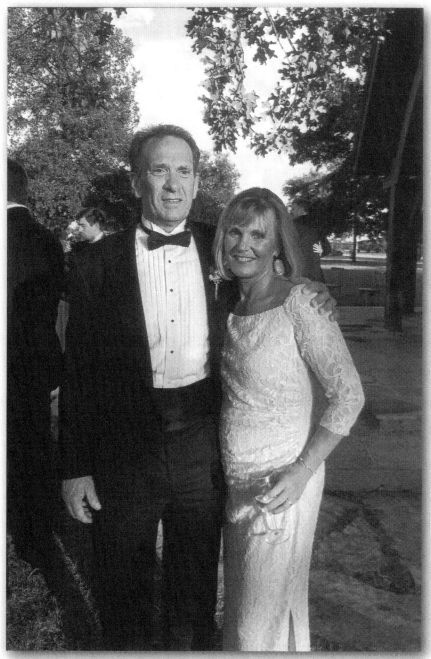

Ted and Pat at Luke and Blake's wedding, 2015

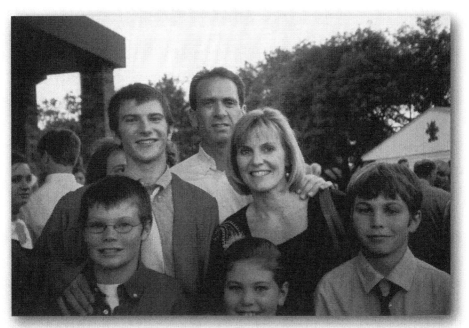

Hinson family at Matt's Bishop Kelley High School graduation, 2004

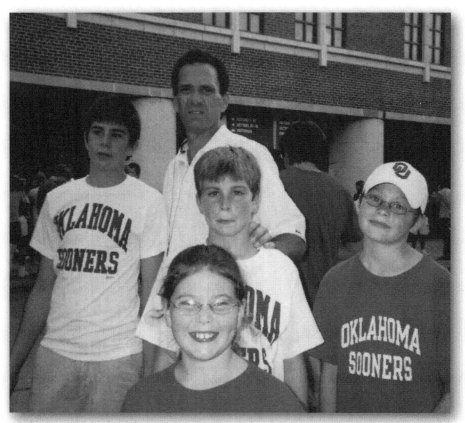

Anna, Luke, Samuel, Daniel, Ted at University of Oklahoma football game, 2004

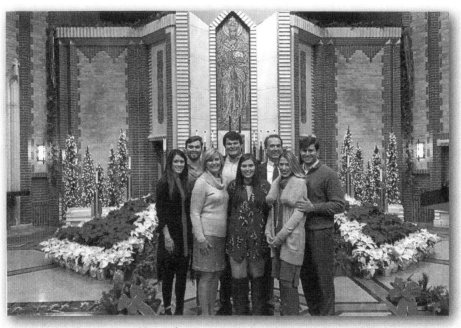

Family Christmas at Christ the King Catholic Church, Tulsa, Oklahoma 2016

Front: Pat, Anna, Blake (Luke's wife),

Back: Shelby Thomas (Samuel's girlfriend), Samuel, Daniel, Ted, Luke

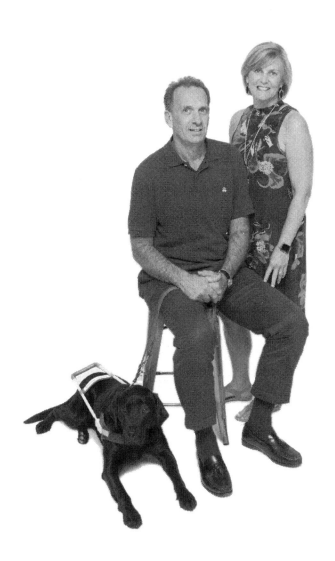

Pat and Ted Hinson with Kansas, 2017

About the Author

Ted Hinson was born and raised in Tulsa, Oklahoma. He attended the University of Oklahoma and then returned to Tulsa in 1987. He and his wife, Pat, raised their five children in the city.

Hinson has worked in the oil and gas industry since graduating from college. In 1986, he unexpectedly lost his sight but was able to continue his successful business career. He and Pat still live in Tulsa, where Hinson is active in many different community groups.

Ted may be contacted through his website, www.tedhinson.com, or by direct email ted@tedhinson.com.

Made in the USA
San Bernardino, CA
05 December 2018